A BIT ABOUT ME

Although this is my first book on herbs. Many know me by my herbal recipes on many sites and blogs as well as face-book. Let me be clear up front, I am not a registered herbalist. I have however worked with herbs my entire life.

I first started at age six (52 years ago) when I started making perfumes from roses and lily of the valley with my mother. Since then I have fanned out to include healthful medicine chest items with "Salves" being my passion.

At the age of seven, I had a series of accidents. All resulted in emergency visits. It was then I was first told I was allergic to almost all modern antibiotics after my last accident that year. I had been bitten by the neighbors dog and the antibiotic (the hospital administered) almost killed me. So you can see there have been many times that my life has literally depended on learning about herbs.

Most my information I learned from my mother as she had from hers -a long line of hedge witches (people who use herbs for healing). Some of my learning has been books, Internet and self discovery. I love learning about herbs I have a unique ability to create recipes simply by knowing the herbs uses. I can do that with regular recipes as well. I am what I call an "off the cuff" recipe creator.

I am by definition a hedge witch, which (for the sake of this book) means I learned it from my Pagan roots (people who have done homemade herbals and have had to count of their knowledge for their family's health).

This book is designed so anyone can use it to create healthful medicine chest items, perfumes and some personal care items. Unlike many other books it also allows you the freedom to check out the herbs and create recipes of your own by giving basic recipe percentages that you can interchange with any herb you want to use to make one of a like creations designed to heal whatever ailment you need to. This book can also be used to start a home business by making these preparations and selling them at craft fairs or on-line. My hope is that people stop counting on so many drugs that create more side effects than they help.

However I need to say for all the Pagans and Wiccans out there, unlike a hedge witches directory, it does "NOT" have magical times or days to pick each herb for magical purposes nor does it tell you what day is best to create your concoctions. It also does "NOT" follow the moon in any way. It is simply an easy to follow basic herbal designed so that anyone can feel at home using for making healthful alternatives to prescription drugs.

If you are a hedge witch or using an herbal magically, you will also need to know that information to produce your herbals. There are many such books out there with that information. This however is NOT one of those.

This book is simply an easy to follow, easy to create, book of information and recipes you will not find anywhere else. Why? Because the recipes are my tried and true recipes from years of using them.

I started sharing recipes on-line almost 10 years ago on a few recipe sights and ran a few groups (9) on a sight that later closed. It quickly became apparent to me that others were also seeking alternatives to prescription drugs without the dangerous side effects). That is why I wrote this book.

So.... lets get started.

~Book of Hedge Witch Herbals~

Notes:
I have used numerous on-line resources from over the last 15 years, personal knowledge taught to me by mother, sister and friends and the following books to complete this book.

Readers digest family guide to natural medicines

National geographic guide to medicinal herbs (Thank you for the interesting notes)

Complete natural medicine guide to 50 common medicinal herbs by Heather Boon, BscPhm, PhD and Michael Smith, BPharm, MR PharmS, ND

If there were only two books I would suggest you pick up and they are "Culpepper's herbal" and an"Audubon Society book of wild plants" from your area. The last book has great pictures and advice for finding plants in the wild.

CHAPTER 1 ~ LETS GET STARTED ~

First let me state, Check with your herbalist, doctor or whatever health care person you trust before using anything new. Also because allergies are usually unknown until they happen, test everything on your inner arm before using it the first time. Give it twenty-four hours then if no side effects (rashes) then precede in using. My advice is start small on doses taken internally and work up.

You can see that both essential oils and herbs are used in this book. However how to make an essential oil wasn't going to be covered because of the amount of work for the product. But as an after thought I decided to at least tell you how to make them and with that recipe you can make any essential oil you wish to make.

So lets do that first.

~MAKING AN ESSENTIAL OIL~

Essential oils are done by steam distilling an herb, a time consuming endeavor. For many, the work vs the yield, will be disheartening But for those who want to know how to do it, here is the equipment you will need.
1 tea kettle (glass preferred or stainless steel)

1 (3-5 foot approximate) hose as close around to the size of the kettles pour spout as possible.

Duct tape or other electrical tape that is heat and water proof to secure the hose to the kettle spout.

A bowl of ice cubes that the hose can pass throw

A large wide jar or clear bowl to catch the steam and essential oil in

A tincture jar with a dropper top

Large handfuls of herbs that produce essential oils (not all do)

distilled water

Attach the hosing to the tea kettle's spout and secure with duct tape.
Run the hose through a bowl of ice at a lower level that the tea kettle on
the stove.
Then on an even lower level (like a chair) place the hose end into the
widemouthed jar and secure it so it doesn't fall out.
Fill the kettle with a heaping handful of herbs and fill with distilled water.
Now when your steam goes into the jar there will be a water level and
on top there will be an oil level.
You will have to refill the water as it gets low and keep an eye on the
water level going into the jar so it doesn't overflow.
Now once it done and is cooled, use the tincture dropper cap to carefully
lift the essential oil from the top of the water (be careful not to pick up
any water) and place it in a small dark glass bottle and recap with the
dropper cap you used to lift the essential oil with.
Label and date.
NOTE: I always add the uses to that label, that way you know at a
glance what it is used for. Trust me once you have a few different
concoctions their uses will blur together unless you use them all the
time.

This book basically how to make salves, compresses, infusions,
decoction's, liniments, tinctures, ointments, tonics and poultices along
with how to make perfumes (chapter 7) and how to dry herbs (chapter
2). I also took the liberty to dissect some "over the counter" natural
medicine chest items. Chapters 5 and 6 are devoted to "Copy Cats".

~OTHER NON HERB INGREDIENTS THAT ARE OR CAN BE USED IN
RECIPES.~

Aloe Vera – inflammation, burns, anti-fungal

Epsom salts – sooths, relieves itching and moisturizes

Sea salt – sooths, moisturizes, vitamins and minerals

Vitamin E – soften, firms, heals, emollient

Vitamin A & D ointment - soften and firms, heals

witch hazel – antioxidant, anti-inflammatory, antiseptic, astringent

Argan oil – reduces wrinkles, loaded with fatty acids, antioxidant

Castor oil – can be taken internally to relieve constipation, used for arthritis, sciatica, back pain, mold inhibitor

Emu oil – Dry skin, hair loss, arthritis, Omega 3, 6, and 9, natural anti-inflammatory, itchy skin, Psoriasis, Eczema, Rosacea

Grape-seed oil – Can be taken internally as well as used in salves and recipes

Jojoba oil – anti-yeast, antibacterial, great for hair, skin

Olive oil (EV)-full of vitamins, a great moisturizer, antibacterial, anti-fungal, hypoallergenic, moisturizes without clogging pores, aids in cell regeneration. Taken internally it lowers LDL (the bad ones) while raising HDL (the good ones).

Sweet Almond oil – locks in moisture, improves skins elasticity

Organic Sunflower oil – loaded with vitamins, can trigger arthritis (so be careful)

Wheatgerm oil – high in minerals and vitamin E used as a preservative, anti-oxidant, great for aging or injured skin

Coconut oil -proven to help heal burns, anti-microbial, anti-viral, anti-bacterial, & a great moisturizer

Bees wax – Can buy in a pound chunk, shredded or in 1 oz bars.
1 (1 oz) bar equals 4 tablespoons. Antibacterial used as a thickening agent in salves, lip balms and lotions. Emulsifier, seals in moisture, preservative

Cocoa butter – Usually sold in jars or push up containers. Antibacterial, anti-fungal, antiseptic, moisturizer

Shea butter – antibacterial, anti-fungal, antiseptic, moisturizer

Clays – green is very drying to skin use for greasy skin, white (Fullers earth) has a very fine texture,

Red clays are loaded with minerals especially iron.

~AND FROM THE KITCHEN WE FIND: ~

Basil relieves headache, makes a great cordial to clean lungs, comforting heart, dispels melancholy.

Cayenne pepper – brings blood to affected area, heat, pain relief

Cornstarch - adsorbs moisture, removes spots

Distilled water – to dilute sprays and perfumes. To make your own distilled water simply fill a pot with water and bring to a boil and low boil ten minutes. Then turn off the heat. Leave it undisturbed until it is cooled (say an hour) and carefully pour the top two thirds into another container. Do not disturb the bottom third of the water. Then you discard the bottom third of the water. The top two thirds is now distilled.

Honey – antibacterial, thickener, moisturizer

Lemon - Anti-tumor, anti-fungal, antibacterial, antiviral, astringent, anti-inflammatory, immune stimulant, diuretic, digestive, expectorant, calming.

Lime - antiseptic, antiviral, astringent, aperitif, bactericidal, disinfectant, restorative

Orange -Antidepressant, antispasmodic, slows digestion, mildly sedative, increase energy, boost the immune system, reduce fever, antibacterial

Thyme – antibiotic used in many tooth pastes, throat gargles, sprays and great for any ailment in the mouth.

Vodka (100 proof) – is used in making tincture or preserving essential oils in tinctures, cordials, tonics, elixirs, sprays and perfumes. NOTE: You can use brandy or even a wine if making a tonic or in making liqueurs cordials elixirs, as well as homemade flavored vodka's.

~ SPECIAL NOTES ~

A fragrance oil is just that - a fragrance. It has no health benefits. They are used for the scent only.

An Essential Oil has health benefits and is used for it's medicinal value as well as fragrance.

NOTE: Do NOT interchange a fragrance oil for an essential oil, but you can exchange a essential oil for a
 fragrance oil.

~ UNDERSTANDING THIS BOOK ~

Compress - a way to deliver a tea to a topical area (skin) by soaking a cloth in a tea then applying to skin usually 10-15 minutes at a time.

Decoction – simmered plant material in water and then drank. Another name for medicinal tea

Essential oil- (also called volatile oil) ahydrophobid, aromatic volatile oil found in specialized glands of most plants. (to make them refer to the first part of this chapter) And read the notes about usage.

Infusion – like decoction it is another word for tea. Herb in boiled water that has sat awhile. In infusion is usually stronger than a decoction.

Infused oil – herb and oil together and usually left 2-3 weeks. Note some require sun some do not. Or it can be heated on warm for 1 hour in a crock pot on on top of stove. Then strained and more herb added and redone. Then strained again and bottled.

Ligament – herb defused in apple cider vinegar usually but also can be infused in other things some do petroleum jelly. NOTE: Warning on petroleum jelly. It is made from petroleum and is flammable.

Poultice – a preparation of fresh crushed plant material that is moistened. Or a chewed plant material, then put onto the skin and covered with a bandage.

Tincture – A concentrate made from herb, flower or root with vodka or brandy

Tonic – made from herbs flowers or roots and made with brandy and is not in a concentrated form.

~OTHER IMPORTANT INFORMATION~

Acetyl-l-carnitine – thwarts off Alzheimer's disease, enhances neurological (brain)transmitters

Adaptogen a substance that strengthens the bodies natural defenses to cure illnesses and protects
 against them.

Aloin -acts as a laxative

EO – essential oil Must be diluted before using.

FO – fragrance oil for perfume dilution is 1/4 oz (2 teaspoons) per 8 oz perfume, or for eye cream 1/3
 teaspoon.

Fluoride – Remember this stuff, the dentist said your kids needed this on their teeth to prevent cavities. Well they lied it actually destroys the teeth's enamel. It is actually a byproduct of strip mining and is toxic. (Way to go US government regulators)

GABA -Interacts with Neurotransmitters and receptors

g – (gram) a unit of measure. There are 28 of them in an ounce.

Hypericin - has been shown to kill the HIV virus. (Doctors never tell you this)

In vitro – transferred to unborn child in womb.

Mucilage – a gelatinous substance found in some plants. Used as a soothing agent.

Oleanolic acid - inhibits bacteria.

Purgative- an agent that relieves constipation.

Rhizome – a elongated root usually horizontal subterranean plant stem thicker by deposits of reserve food material, that produces shoots above and roots below, different than the true root by having buds, nodes, and usually scale like leaves. This is the root you would use to create a tincture from a root.

Silicin – acts like aspirin to relieve pain.

Triterpenoid – antioxidant (reduces oxygen radical damage)

Zinc oxide – mildly antiseptic, anti-fungal, antibacterial, and blocks UVA rays and UVB Radiation. Used in diaper rash, sunblock and kills most things that try to live on your body (scabies, crabs)

~USEFUL Conversions~

1 oz bar of beeswax equals 4 tablespoons

1 teaspoon of essential oil equals 25 drops.

2 tablespoons are in 1 oz.

1/4 cup liquid equals 4 tablespoons or 2 oz

5 ml equals 1 teaspoon

15 ml equals 1 tablespoon

30 ml equals an oz

~ DILUTING ESSENTIAL OILS (to use on your body)~

NOTE: In recipes essential oils are diluted by other ingredients in a recipe, anywhere that you see essential oil it will be undiluted unless it says pacifically in carrier oil. To use on your body without putting it into a recipe you need to dilute the oil with a carrier oil.

A carrier oil is used to dilute essential oils.

Basic recipe used as a preservative 6 drops per ounce of cream or oil or 1/3 teaspoon per cup of cream or oil.

THEY INCLUDE

Grape-seed oil can be used on body but not hair.

Jojoba oil Usually used in hair products, said to help restore natural color.

Extra virgin olive oil can be used for your body or hair

Sweet Almond oil if making an ear oil but can be used for anything.

Sunflower oil used in tinctures, rubs, salves

Basic preservative measurements for antioxidants A,C,E

IN EVERY 8 OUNCE CREAM OR OIL ADD ANY OF THE FOLLOWING
1/4 teaspoon vitamin A powder
1 teaspoon vitamin C powder
1 teaspoon Vitamin E

A STANDARD RECIPE TO DELUTE AN ESSENTIAL OIL TO USE DIRECTLY
ON SKIN IS
1 oz carrier oil
5 drops essential oil

~ THINGS YOU SHOULD CONCIDER BUYING~
(Not a good idea to use cooking   items interchangeably due to some
products shouldn't go into your mouth.)

A small sauce pan for melting things on the stove. Pick either stainless
or glass because essential oils leach. Or do as I do and use the next item
for that.

A 1-2 cup glass measuring cup To melt things in the microwave and
measure with.

A mini crock pot (to infuse oils and butters if you don't wish to use the
stove top)

Spoons to measure, tablespoon and teaspoon

A separate set of beaters for a hand mixer.

A coffee grinder for roots and herbs (Your best purchase if using roots or
barks

A few different sized glass bowls to mix in (very small to large- do not
use same bowls as you eat out of)

Glass Jars and bottles – so start collecting.

Any dark colored glass pint alcohol bottles (great for ligaments, large
volume tinctures and rubs especially if you are preparing ahead for a
craft show)

Qt mason jars

Pint mason jars

Jelly jars

Any small glass jar with tight fitting lid.

THESE ARE SOME I ESPECIALLY LIKE:

Orman's Horseradish sauce (a 7 oz square jar with a black top. Best part is every logo comes off with a finger nail. Very good for large salves and bath salts

Star-bucks Iced coffee in a 11 oz glass bottle. All the writing also can be removed with a finger nail. Great for shampoos, cream rinses, bubble baths, and alright for tonics. Also good for storing large volume tinctures if you are making craft fair item's (make sure if a tincture that it is kept in the dark.)

Pint liquor pint bottles. They come in a variety of colors from smoked glass to green and blue. (as do wine bottles). I use then for tonics and homemade liqueurs.

Pint sized mayonnaise jars, the glass ones.

SPECIAL NOTES:

Many of the chain stores have some wonderful lip salve jars. The one that starts with a "W" has them 2 for $0.88 in the sample isle of the toiletries dept. They come in blue, yellow, green, and pink. They are very useful for not only lips products but recipes like the acne overnight cream recipe, lips salves and shimmers, age defying cream, eye creams and as sample jars if making stocking stuffer's or craft show offers and door prizes. They look so pretty that they will bring people over to see what you have. You can color coordinate lip salves to condense that way,. Like green for mint, thyme or other green herb, pink for flower herbs, yellow for calendula, honeysuckle, or any lemon product, blue for maybe coffee flavored or blueish flower preparations as well as kids lip balms (blueberry, blue-moon, blue cotton candy.

Also at all the dollar stores have an assortment of plastic spray bottles, flip top squeeze bottles and perfume bottles. Many have lotion bottles or travel packs of empty container.

You would be surprised how lovely an antique spray perfume bottle can be filled with a signature fragrance that you made yourself.

Remember essential oils will leach into plastic over time. So try for glass whenever possible or discard after a couple of weeks.

When I first started I had every one I knew saving all glass containers. I also bought every Mason jar I could find at garage sales, the salvation army, good will and any of the real sale shops. Which is also a great place to acquire antique perfume bottles or glass containers.

Chapter 2 HERBS

Herbs are easy to grow and so rewarding. Once started, they grow year after year minimizing the cost of creating healthful alternatives to over the counter drugs. Check the Chapter 3 for wild herbs around you and you might find some free medicinal herbs around your yard.

This book only contains a partial list of herbs that are used medicinally, but it will get you started. They are the most widely used ones as least as far as I am concerned.

~ TO DRY HERBS ~

There are two very good ways to dry herbs. The one best suited will depend on the herb you are drying.

Type 1: Gather in a small bunch and hang upside down in a cool well ventilated place. Some do closets and some hang in kitchens. Ventilation is most important because of chance of mold. For that reason basements are not preferable. Attics in the late fall work well if you add a gentle fan.

Type 2: Some herbs because of their delicate nature or seeds it is best to lightly attach tissue paper around them. You can do this by sewing thread ties on 4 sides and attaching it to the bundle. Don't draw it tightly, just allow to hang around it.

An alternative is to lay a split opened paper bag or tissue paper under the herb. I found those are better laid out on a screen. You can buy actual drying screens at any grow or hydro shop. They cost around $30.

You can also make your own from screening and a wooden homemade frame. If you are not mechanically incline you can simply buy a screen ready made to fit an imaginary window and suspend it between two milk crates. That is a great way to make multiple levels of drying racks, Just stack them as high as you wish. Then put a fan in the room (not directly blowing in the herbs) and you are set.

Dry roots by hanging like mullein with a string or on screens. Sun drying roots is quite popular. You can use dental floss, regular sewing thread, or even fishing line to hang with.

Mullein deserves special mention here as it is a unique plant. As a child I used to pick it and feel it's soft furry thick leaves. (Just so you know there are three fuzzy plants that could be in your backyard, mullein is just one of them.) It feels like an expensive sweater. My father used to call it the "butt wipe plant", saying it was soft enough to wipe your bottom with if you were camping in the wild. Due to their thick furry leaves either dry on racks or by threading them spaced apart and hanging the string like a banner with the leaves spaced apart about an inch in between (I do it this way). Remember it is an unusual plant and is best harvested in the spring when it is just coming up and not the fall like most plants. Take only the small new leaves before they get to regular size They have the most health benefits.

NOTE: If any of your herbs develops mold, toss them.

I have heard some people dry herbs in a dehydrator. Some health values can be lost through heating. If you intend to use a dehydrating your herbs you should use the lowest setting possible. My thought is use those herbs as spices and not medicines.

In warm wet seasons I have had to use a dehumidifier in the room along with fans (not placed on the herb but so the air moves in the room).

THIS IS THE MEANS (IN THIS BOOK) THAT I WILL USE TO ALLERT YOU TO A HERBS SPECIAL BEHAVIORS BELOW

Herbs / part used / qualities /side effects

No know side effects - A

Allergies are rare - B

Safe in taken in reasonable amounts - C

Warning - D

~ HERBS LIST ~

NOTE: Just because you do not see a medication you are taking in the list of do not take, it is wisest to check with your doctor before taking the herb especially if your medication is used for the same purpose as the do not take list.

ALOE - inside leaf– Compounds (polysaccharides, aloin(acts as a laxative) enzymes)- anti-viral, anti-inflammatory, antibacterial, anti tumor, anti-viral, anti fungal- osteoarthritis, Psoriasis, sunburn, irritable bowel syndrome, lowers blood sugar levels in type 2 diabetes, speeds healing of diabetic wounds, reduces risk of infection, hemorrhoids, insomnia, headaches, gum diseases, kidney ailments, the latex (outer shell of leaf) is prescribed for constipation, externally softens and restores skin tissue, burns, sores, radiation burns, diabetic sores, blemishes, dandruff, psoriasis, used after dental procedures– (gel) internally ulcers, stomach disorders – B - NOTE: dried aloe latex not discussed in this book. INTERESTING NOTE: a medical document found in ancient Egypt called the "Codex Ebers" dating back to 1552 BC mentions Aloe Vera.- D. PRECAUSIONS: Although it heals, it is not good for deep wounds or after surgery (not sure why) If pregnant, small kids and those with severe
gastrointestinal symptoms should not take it internally.

ARNICA – entire plant including the roots – Compounds (sesquiterpene Lactones) – Anti-inflammatory, bruises, muscle soreness, back pain, strains, sprains, arthritis, rheumatic pain, swelling from fractures
or injuries, acne, chapped lips, eases pain – D. Warning: Do not take internally (can cause Heart arrhythmias or respiratory collapse. Do not use on broken skin-
INERESTING NOTE: Arnica means "lambskin". Arnica was it's effects were first published in "Commentarii in sex libros Pedacii Dioscorides" a botanical masterpiece and published in 1544 AD.

ANISE – seeds- coughs, digestion, gas, increasing milk production in nursing mothers, aphrodisiac, for colic, nausea – taken internally as tea
-
A.

ASH – Leaves, bark, fruit – Quinine like properties Dropsy, Rheumatism, snake bites, used as a replacement for Peruvian bark, used in decoction, tinctures or tonic - D. Warning: take in moderation

BASIL – leaf, volatile oils - coughs, expel worms, in snuff to relieve headaches, stomach cramps, constipation, vomiting – taken internally as tea or as a syrup for coughs – A.

BILBERRY (blueberry) - berries, leaf- compounds (arthrocyanosides, Tannins) – antioxidant, astringent, anti-inflammatory, circulation, varicose veins, eye health, preserves brain function, nausea, vomiting, hypertension, diabetes, bladder infections, atherosclerosis, venous insufficiency, eye sight, diarrhea, age related degeneration diseases, heart health, colon cancer, cancer tumors.-A.

BIRCH – inter bark and trigs into infusions, birch bud into essential oil- salicylic acid (active ingredient in aspirin), tannic acid,- anti- inflammatory, astringent, antiviral, antiseptic, tissue healing, INTERESTING NOTE: Also cuts grease

BLACK COHOSH – root (Rhizome) – compound phytoestrogen (natural estrogen)- diuretic, considered a womans herb, drank to relieve menopause, menstrual cramps, Algonquin Indians use it for kidney problems, and the Cherokee use it for fatigue, tuberculosis. Iroquois apply it externally to relieve joint pain. Hot flashes, night sweats, vaginal dryness, premenstrual discomforts, irritability, mood swings, anxiety, arthritis, melancholy - A.D. WARNING in a few cases minor gastrointestinal upset has occurred. In rare cases liver damage has been reported. Suggest you check with Doctor if you have liver problems before taking this herb.

BLACK HAW (also called Cramp bark)- bark – compounds (beta- adrenergic receptors, salicin (related to aspirin)) -anti spasmodic, bark, stem and root (fruit can be eaten and used in jams and wine) bark used in tea for menstrual cramps, prevent miscarriage, and calms uterine spasms afterbirth, muscle spasms, small pox, fever, regulate menstrual flow, uterine prolapse, morning sickness, heaving menstrual bleeding, asthma, lowering blood pressure, digestive and urinary cramping, Used by mid-wives following a birth or to prevent miscarriage – A, D. WARNING do not use during pregnancy with out a doctors advice

BONESET – leaves and flowering tops - relieves break-bone fever (from a strain of influenza virus), digestion, malaria, and snakebite, fevers from cold and flu, break up mucus – C.

BURDOCK ROOT (stems can be eaten) – volatile oil, Compounds (insulin, polyacetylenes, arctiopicrin, Alkaloids, silicon)- antimicrobial, diuretic, anti-tumor, rheumatoid arthritis, indigestion, kidney trouble, dropsy, high fevers, gout, leprosy, dandruff, acne, skin conditions, hair stimulant, brewed as a tonic as a diuretic, blood purifier, mild laxative – D. warning do not take if pregnant, or have diabetes, allergies can include a worsening of symptoms. Drug interactions oral hypoglycemis agents

BUTTERBUR (other names Plague flower, Woodland umbrella plant, blatter-dock)- leaves -(grow in marshy ground) – weak heart, used as a tonic for dropsy, fevers, disinfectant (plagues and pestilence) used in cordials, a appetite stimulant, whooping cough, asthma, migraines, headache, pain, stomach ulcers, hay fever, irritable bowel – D. warning: Some butterbur products may contain pyrrolizidine alkaloids (PAS) do not take those internally. Make your own to avoid that.

BUTTERWORT – leaves – mucilage, tannins, benzoic acid, gum, and enzyme - antispasmodic, sedative, purgative, diuretic, blood pressure, used to coagulate milk, hair dye (golden yellow)

CALENDULA (pot marigold)- flowers, whole plant used in tinctures Triterpenoid compounds (oleanolic acid - (helps it seal over with new tissue))- anti-inflammatory, antioxidant, antibacterial, emollient, dermatitis, wounds, skin problems, eczema, psoriasis, varicose veins, abscesses, acne, skin abrasions, wounds, kill bacteria, gum inflammation, gingivitis, breast radiation (use this in place of Trolamine), dermatitis from radiation, blond highlights in hair – B. Those allergic to the asteraceae family can develop a sensitivity to topical use INTERESTING NOTE: The "1477 Macer's Herbal "claims this herb draws out tumors. In 1699 "Countrie Farme" notes it improves eye sight, headaches, jaundice, and ague (no idea what that publication is maybe a magazine or a news paper). In 1860 it is used by field doctors in civil war to Staunch (stop) bleeding.

CAMPHOR– used in the past for embalming, increasing heat in body, stimulant, sedative (lowers circulation)- D warning – Do not over use and limit quantities as it can numb and if overused paralyze.

CAT'S CLAW – dried inter stem bark (takes plant 3-8 years in order to be old enough to harvest) -compounds(oxindote alkaloids, glycosides) anti-oxidant, anti-inflammatory, asthma, arthritis, rheumatism, cancer, AIDS, a powerful immune system stimulator, rheumatoid arthritis, HIV, Fibromyalgia, chronic fatigue, shingles, mononucleosis, osteoarthritis, ulcers, neuralgia, gastritis, urinary track infections, kidney problems, fevers, intestinal ailments, gonorrhea, birth control – D. WARNING: Do not take if taking an auto-immune suppressant or blood pressure medications. Do not take if under 3 years old, pregnant or nursing – B. side effects can include upset stomach, dizziness, or headaches. If taking for HIV or Cancer do so under a doctors supervision- INTERESTING NOTE: until the 1970's was only know in the amazon as an herbal.

CATNIP – Leaves – sleep aide, menstrual pain, sooths nerves, insect repellent, headache taken internally and externally – A.

CAYENNE– fruit – Compound (Capsaicin) Anti-inflammatory, reduces itching, digestive aide, toothache, ward of chills from a cold, Pain relief, nerve pain, rheumatoid arthritis, osteoarthritis, Fibromyalgia, shingles, post surgical pain, circulation, relieves heartburn, When used in ointments it confuses neurotransmitters in the skin and disrupts pain signals – A. D WARNING: use gloves when working with or applying creams or ointments. Do not get in eyes or soft inter folds of body as it burns. DO NOT apply to broken skin – B.- allergic reactions can include rash, swelling and burning sensations.

CHAMOMILE (Roman or German)– flowers – Volatile oil, compounds (apigenin, tannins, flavonoids) -mild sedative, anti-inflammatory, antiseptic, astringent, antioxidant, antimicrobial, anti-allergenic, nervous tension, muscle cramps, skin conditions, combats insomnia, inflammation Extract), heals wounds (Extract), dissolves kidney and gallstones, infant colic, Cohn's disease, digestion, heartburn, diarrhea, muscle tension, eczema, inflamed skin, gastritis, menstrual cramps, prevents wrinkles, good moisturizing, flatulence, irritable bowel syndrome, acute stomach upset. A. B. Rare cases severe ragweed allergies can trigger an allergy, also do not take if allergic to the asteraceae family.

CHICKWEED - Herb – Volatile oil – Used for malnutrition, rheumatism, cramps, palsy, possible help for paralysis (in minute doses), Asthma, wounds, peritonitis, internal inflammation – D. Taken internally in large doses produces a static condition. Interesting Note: The star like flowers open at 9 if the weathers fine and remains open for 12 hours.

CLEAVERS(goose-grass) Grows wild in US- leaves infused or crushed)- glyosides, tannin, citric acid – anti-cancer, purifies the blood, appetite suppressant, astringent, diuretic, detoxifies, psoriasis, can be used on cats for FLUDT, cleanses the lymph system and skin diseases, lowers blood pressure without lowering heart rate. Is also a coffee substitute (Use roasted seeds)

COMFREY – leaves, roots- allantoin (repairs damaged tissue) tannins, saponins, alkaloids (toxic to liver and carcingenic)- anti wrinkle, repairs damaged skin, stimulates new skin growth, heals wounds, dandruff, varicose veins- D Do not boil comfrey as it destroys the allantoin, do not take internally and if pregnant use sparingly on skin.

CREEPING WINTERGREEN (Teaberry) American Indians use it for breathing while moving heavy loads, aches and pains, analgesic, anti-inflammatory, aromatic, astringent, carminative, diuretic, emmenagogue (an agent that hastens menstrual flow), stimulant and tonic. An infusion of the leaves is used to relieve flatulence and colic. ESSENTIAL OIL is used for rheumatism, sciatica, myalgia, sprains, neuralgia and catarrh. The oil is sometimes used in the treatment of cellulitis, a bacterial infection that causes the skin to become inflamed - D. WARNING: Do NOT overuse essential oil eternally can cause liver or kidney damage

DANDELION – leaves, root (as medicine) flowers as tea and eat – Terpenes, phytosterois, insulin, potassium) -diuretic, hypoglycemia, liver, kidney and gall bladder problems, diuretic, appetite stimulant, digestion, mild laxative, dyspepsia, loss of appetite, leaves water retention– B. dermatitis

Echinacea (also known as purple coneflower, Kansas or Missouri snakeroot)– root (usually), Leaves – compounds (polydaccharides, glycoporoteins, alkyl amides) caffeic acid derivatives (enchinacoside, cichoric, cynarin)- Anti-inflammatory, antibacterial, anti-allergenic, toothache, snake bite, insect bites, heals wounds, toothache, sore gums, coughs, respiratory infections, fevers, fights viruses, stimulates white blood cells, skin conditions, fights infection, stimulates immune system, eases colds and sore throats, diabetes mellitus, lupus, HIV/AIDES, rheumatoid arthritis, burns, athletics foot– B. D. WARNING: If allergic to the daisy family do not take. It is rare but can result in asthma attack, anaphylaxis, or urticaria. Also do not use with the following medications: Itraconazole, lovastin, and fexofenadine. Also check with Doctor if taking Birth control pills. High doses can cause nausea. If allergic to ragweed do not take Echinacea internally.

Elder – berries, Flowers– Compounds (Vitamin C, sambucol, sterols, triterpenes, phenolic acids flavonoids)- anti-viral, Purgative, antioxidant, fight infections, anti-inflammatory, rheumatic aches, sprains, wounds, bruises, coughs, colds, skin conditions, sinus and nasal, congestion, sneezing and itching associated with allergies, immune enhancer, bronchitis INTERESTING FACTS: most uses magically for any tree, Put in the US Pharmacopoeia from 1820 -1831 then was dropped - D. WARNING: Some elders are poisonous. European Elder and S. Nigar Var. Canadensis Both have editable fruit. C.D. CAUSION: if you have an autoimmune condition, consult Doctor. Eating unripe fruit or any part of the rest of the plant can cause, dizziness, confusion, diarrhea, vomiting, nausea. No drug interactions have been found. WARNING Do NOT take if pregnant or nursing. Prolonged use is not recommended.

EUCALYPUS – leaves – Compounds (volatile oils, cineole (eucalyptol)) – expectorant, anti-viral, antibacterial, anti-inflammatory, healing, clears sinuses, sooths mucus membranes, used in toothpaste, balms, mouth washes, throat lozenges, clears sinuses, sore muscles, dandruff, chapped
skin, lower blood sugar (careful diabetics), can be used to lower steroid doses if taken 3 times a day, emphysema, asthma, colds, flu, cough,- D. WARNING: Keep out of eyes

EVENING OF PRIMROSE– seed - asthmatic coughs, stomach problems, neuralgia, whooping cough -A. Evening of primrose essential oil-Adults take 2-8 grams a day- taken in divided doses- seed- oil(fatty acid GLA) atopic asthma (asthma from allergies), atopic eczema, migraines, premenstrual syndrome, anti blood clotting, promotes weight loss, lowers cholesterol and lowers blood pressure, diabetic Neuropathy, endometriosis, mastalgia, psoriasis, rheumatoid arthritis, multiple sclerosis, Sjogren's syndrome, inhibit platelet aggression, schizophrenia, hyperactivity, dementia, Chronic fatigue syndrome, alcoholism, renal disease, cancer, obesity– A.

FENNEL– seed – volatile oil 8%(anethole)- anti-inflammatory, expectorant, ayurvedic, increases milk supply in lactating women, appetite suppressant, decreases food cravings, buffers laxatives cramping effects, freshens breath, sooths sore throats, heals infected gums, calms stomachaches, used for some cancers, aides in digestion, taken in tea it stimulates appetite in anorectics, menstrual cramps, used in a gargle for sore throat and bad breath, gas and bloating, a tea relieves coughs and sore throats -A.

FENUGREEK – seed- oil 40% (mucilage)- used in treating skin irritations and wounds, tonic to ease stomach ailments, tuberculosis, bronchitis, sore throats, diabetes, anemia, rickets, expectorant, a laxative, fevers, and waning sexual drive -A.

FEVERFEW – leaf- compound (parthenolide) -any hot inflammation or swelling, anti-fungal, menstrual cramps, arthritis, migraine headache pain and the nausea and vomiting that accompanies them, insect bites, insect repellent, digestion, rheumatoid arthritis. Chew 2-3 leaves. Daily use is most effective. - B. Mouth sores have been reported in a few but go away with repeated use. Also post-Feverfew syndrome (nervousness, tension, fatigue, joint pain). D. Warning: don't take if pregnant, nursing or under 2 years old. Interaction with drug Warfarin
Added information: For pain leaves used in tincture, tea, or pill. As an anti-inflammatory use flowering tops

GINGER- under ground lateral root rhizome- compounds (shogaois, Gingerois) – antimicrobial, migraines, digestion, nausea from pregnancy, all the arthritis's, colds, nausea, seafood poisoning, an oil massage alleviates spinal and joint problems, nausea from anesthesia, inhibits platelet aggression, myalgia's, used for recouping from illnesses, a mild stimulant, circulation, motion sickness, burn pain -A.

GINKGO BILOBA – leaf- compounds (glycosides, biotides terpene lactones, triterpenes, diterpenes) increases peripheral circulation (dilate arteries, veins, and capillaries) Raymaud's syndrome, dementia, increases blood flow to the brain (used in senility, short tern memory loss), sores, diarrhea, vertigo, cerebral insufficiency, impotence, bronchial, asthmatic and pulmonary conditions, tinnitus, vascular diseases, improves mental functions -A. D. drug interaction: do not take if taking "Theoretical"

GINGSING (American - Canadian)– root- compounds (panaxans, phytrochemicals)- antioxidant, hot flashes, blood glucose, hemoglobin, anti-inflammatory, adaptogen, stress and fatigue, hypertension, hyperglycemia, stimulates blood flow, strengthens immune systems especially in elderly, nervous system, controls type 1 diabetes, stimulant, reduces cholesterol, protects against certain types of cancer, mental clarity - B. some experience stomach upset or headache. D. WARNING monitor your blood pressure while taking this herb. CAUSION IF: Acute illness, premenstrual women with unstable period cycles, controlled diabetes, use of stimulants.

GOLDENSEAL -root (rhizomes) - alkaloids (hydrastine, berberine, canadine, hydrastinine) Antiseptic, antimicrobial, wound healing, cleanses the liver and blood, restores digestive functions in alcoholics, colds and flu, hay fever, vaginitis, sinusitis, canker sores, diarrhea, conjunctivitis, sore throat, Cherokees use it for sore eyes, mouth ulcers, tuberculosis, edema, extracts are used for multiple strains of helicobacter pylori (a bacteria that is responsible for most of peptic ulcers and gastric cancers) – C-D caution if pregnant can cause contractions, hypertension – INTERESTING NOTE: the US regulated it twice in history 1830-1840 and 1865-1936. And was an official drug from 1830 to 1959. Due to its highly bitter taste it is not recommended as a tea with honey.

HATHORN – leaf, flowers, fruit- Compounds (Triterpene glycosides, oligomeric procyanidins) -treat heart ailments, dilates blood vessels, lowers blood pressure, strengthens the heart, mild sedative, congestive heart failure, heart pain, diuretic, sore throat, high cholesterol, removes build up of fatty plaque in blood vessels, atherosclerosis, maintains normal heart rhythm, improves blood flow through heart, heart arrhythmia - D. WARNING: Pregnancy or lactating, heart medications. INTERESTING FACT: People with left ventricle damage (the left ventricle muscle of the heart is the hardest working as it pumps blood from the heart and throughout the body) this herb will significantly reduce the risk of sudden cardiac death from 12 to 24 months

HORSE CHESTNUT also called buckeyes (do not confuse with editable chestnuts or the candy)- seeds and bark (not fruit)– compound (asecin) - anti-inflammatory, varicose veins, blood clots, arthritis, nocturnal leg cramps, phlebitis, joint pains, diarrhea, hemorrhoids, improves vein elasticity, used by native Americans to ease pain and inflammation of hemorrhoids, -D. pregnancy, lactating, kidney or liver disease. Drug interaction with diabetic and anti-coagulation drugs.

HORSETAIL – infused leaves- silica- antioxidant, anti-inflammatory,kidney and bladder stones, incontinence, bladder infections, tuberculous, jaundices, hepatitis, weak bones, frostbite, weight loss, hemorrhage, wounds and burns, gout, strengthens nails and hair' INTERESTING NOTE: it is also used as an abrasive in cleaning medal and wood.

HYSSOP – herb - Volatile oils, hyssopin, tannin, flavone glycosides, marrubin- Internally used for respiratory ailments, expectorant, speed digestion of fat, relieves gas, Externally is used for treating sores, used in liquors – A.

JUNIPER– berry – Volatile oil, tannin, terpene, juniperin, ascorbic acid – disinfectant, anti-inflammatory, diuretic, antiseptic, expectorant, congestion, coughs, psoriasis, intestinal ailments, urinary track infections, joint pain, ulcers, wounds, high fevers, respiratory infections, stimulates appetite, chronic arthritis, diuretic, stimulates uterine contraction, stomachache, colds, genitourinary infections including cystitis – D. WARNING do NOT take if pregnant as it can start contractions. Do NOT take over 6 weeks of you have weak or damaged Kidneys. Although it is used for a range of kidney ailments it is not for kidney infections. Interesting note: in a study with animals it is an abortfacient (a substance that causes abortions), so do not use internally if pregnant. Avoid this herb if on a hypoglycemic or diuretic therapy.

LAVENDER – flowers- Volatile oils, tannins, flavonoids coumarins)- Antibiotic, antimicrobial, anti-viral, calming, Pain relief, antiseptic, relieves stuffy nose, settles upset stomach, stimulates bile flow, good for liver and gall bladder problems – A.

LEMON BALM (Melissa)– the aerial parts (above ground) – Volatile oil, tannins, rosmarinic acid, polyphenols – anti-spasmodic, sedative, anti-emetic, caminative, anti-microbial, anti-hormonal, diaphoretic, heart conditions, memory, depression, wounds, digestion, anxiety, calms, Alzheimer's, dementia, pediatric conditions, cardiac conditions, insomnia, ADHD, hyperthyroid, cold sores from herpes simplex labialis, headaches, colic, fever blisters, blocks the herpes simplex virus. Eases bloating and gas depression, anxiety, (used in furniture polish, sedative, induces perspiration, relieves fever from colds and flu, menstrual cramps, headache and nerves- A. B. Check with doctor if you have a per-existing thyroid condition, to check on any thyroid medicines you are on. D. WARNING: Check thyroid medicines for possible trouble.

MARSHMALLOW ROOT – root – compound (mucilage) – anti-inflammatory -Internally relieves sore throat, coughs, bronchitis, urinary track infections, colitis, eases constipation, sooths inflamed throat tissues, externally used to sooth skin abrasions- A.

MEADOWSWEET – the aerial parts (above ground)- Volatile oils, flavonoids, tannins, salicylic acid, salicin (aspirin qualities) - anti-inflammatory, analgesic, digestive upset, hyper-acidity, nausea, pediatric diarrhea, relieves arthritis pain, anti-coagulant, decreases frequency of squamous cell carcinoma of the cervix and vagina, used as an ointment in the regression of cervical dysplasia D. WARNING - avoid if pregnant or lactating, asthmatic, diabetes, gout, kidney or liver disease.

MILKTHISTLE – seed, flowering head- compound (silymarin)- anti-oxidant, internally -liver tonic, digestion, stimulates the production of milk, liver disease, cirrhosis, hepatitis, protects against some liver toxins, increases the livers function and regenerates the liver, psoriasis, stimulates cell
production, antidote to deadly death-cap mushroom (the mushroom destroys liver cells but milk thistle extract must be given intravenously) in vitro: anti-coagulant - A. D. Possible warning may interfere with indinavir therapy in patients infected with HIV. Also do not take as a tea.

MULLEIN – leaves, flowers - Compound (Mucilage)- anti-inflammatory, antibacterial, Internally heals, expectorant, demulcent (coats tissues), sooths inflamed membranes, sore throat, chest cold, hoarseness – externally relieves burns, arthritic joints, astringent, respiratory troubles, heals open wounds, bronchitis, asthma, coughs, soothe irritated membranes, yellow mullein flowers in oil relieves ear infections, heal wounds, tuberculosis cough, heal sores, laryngitis, tonsillitis, whooping cough, influenza,- A. D. WARNING: do not use seeds. INTERESTING NOTE: In ancient Rome flower stocks were dipped in hot fat, then dried and used as torches. Later they were used magically and called hag tapers.

MUGWORT– Leaves, root – anti-epileptic, colic, diarrhea, worm infestation, persistent vomiting, sedative, liver tonic, circulation, induces or increases clairvoyance, affects pineal gland, convulsions in children, Keeps away moths, remedy for excessive opium smoking, helps with burn scars, fatigue, trouble sleeping, irregular periods – D. WARNING: may stimulate uterus so do not take internally if pregnant. INTERESTING NOTE: Used by many magicians on eve of St. John.

MYRRH – gum resin- volatile oil and used as food flavoring- astringent, antiseptic, bed sores, heals, cleanses, used in mouthwashes and gargles, sore throat, gingivitis, sore gums, mosquito repellent when burned – A.

NETTLE (stinging nettle) – leaves, rhizome(divided in autumn) - compounds (large amount of chlorophyll, lignans, polysaccharides, lectins, histamine, acetylcholine,)- diuretic, anti-inflammatory,

Revive"s lost mobility (in paralysis or loss of motor functions), Blood purifier, astringent, eczema, skin problems, arthritis, gout, hair loss, prostate, hay fever, rheumatism, paralysis, sciatica, bursitis, osteoarthritis, reduces the sneezing and itching of hay fever, strains, sprains, stimulates milk flow in lactating women, Benign Pro-static hyperplasia (BPH) in men, eczema, psoriasis, chronic skin problems, used for convalescence, Interesting note: if you allow the sting leaves to touch the arthritic or sore joint it counter acts the pain almost instantly and is used by Physicians in Germany. It confuses pain signals to the brain. The oil can be burned like paraffin as candles A-D. WARNING: Do not take if pregnant, Possible drug interactions with diabetes medicines and diuretic medicines when using the root. Skin rashes usually occur if using fresh leaves on skin. Instead use dried leaves, and use dried in capsules for internal use. (In vitro: hypertensive, hypoglycemic, nervous system depressor)

ORRIS ROOT (Iris Rhizome) – Root – Mild diuretic, anti-inflammatory, sinus headaches, Blood-purifier, gland-stimulator, increasing kidney activity, appetite, digestion, and bile flow. Headache, toothaches, muscle and joint pain, migraine, constipation, diabetes, skin disease, bronchitis, colds, cancer, sciatica, inflammation of the spleen. It is also used to cause vomiting, empty the bowels, and promote calmness. Orris root is sometimes applied directly to the affected area for teething, tumors, scars, muscle and joint pain, burns, and cuts, used in sour throat medicines, used in perfumes to combine scents, used often in violet perfumes as it also smells like violets.

PEPPERMINT – leaf- distilled oil, compound (menthol) -antispasmodic, antibacterial, antimicrobial, anti-fungal, anti-viral, antiseptic, hiccups, sea serpent stings, dog bite, rabies, upper respiratory conditions, bronchial conditions, colic, stomachache, mild sedative, muscle and nerve pain, gas, headache, nausea, scabies, spastic colon dyspepsia, irritable bowel syndrome-A. D. WARNING Do not use internally if you have GERD. Infants and young children, achlorhydria (low stomach acid)

PSYLLIUM – seed- seed is dietary fiber (in metamucil), ayurvudic medicine, laxative, inflammatory bowel disease, irritable bowel syndrome, hemorrhoids, lowers blood cholesterol (LDL) when used with diet, heart health, diarrhea, improves insulin resistance to decrease diabetic risk, controlling weight, also in these Kellogg cereals - heart wise and brand buds. D. WARNING: over use will cause diarrhea.

RED RASPBERRY– leaves – compound (tannins)- astringent, woman's tonic, (Fruit) eaten in large quantities is a laxative, increases sweating, eases rheumatism, indigestion. (Leaf used as tea) gargle, sore mouth and throat. Applied to skin cleans wounds, skin ulcers. Regulates menstruation, decreases heavy menstrual flow, Used in pregnancy to strengthen, tone and relax uterus muscle, shorten labor, ease delivery, a decoction is used to tighten teeth when they are loose – A. D. See special note in wild herbs, WARNING: decreases absorption of calcium and magnesium

RHODIOLA (also called gold root or rose root)– rhizome – compounds (rosavin, salidroside) - adaptogen, stimulate, increases serotonin levels, stress, anxiety, depression, fatigue, improves endurance /strength / stamina, enhances attention span, chronic fatigue syndrome, increases mental performance- A.D. WARNING: Do not take if pregnant or taking an anti-depressant drug.

ROSEMARY- leaves, volatile oil contains camphor, compound (flavoniods)- stimulant, stomach upset, digestive disorders, headache, rejuvenates circulatory and nervous systems, used to prevent baldness- C.

SAGE – leaves- oil contains (thujone, cineol, camphor) – astringent, antibacterial, tonsillitis, reduces perspiration, dries sores and mucus, cancer, bronchitis, mouth sores, cleans teeth, sores, colds, fevers, epilepsy, constipation, increases fertility, coughs, respiratory infections, indigestion, purify the blood, whitens yellow teeth when chewed, headaches, congestion, slows dementia, menopausal symptoms, improves memory, gastrointestinal troubles – D. WARNING: Can reduce milk in lactating women, do not take except as flavoring in food if pregnant, Prolonged use of sage oil can cause convulsions. Drug interaction with hormonal therapy

SAW PALMENTTO – berries – volatile oils, fixed oils, compounds (liposterolic, polisaccharides) enzymes (5 alpha-reductase (affects estrogen and progesterone, stops prostate growths) -expectorant, anti-inflammatory, antiseptic, urinary tract disorders (especially in males), libido, enlarged prostate, dysentery, benign pro-static hyperplasia (BPH), Chronic pelvis pain syndrome (CPPS) in men, inflammation of the urethra, bladder disorders, gallstones, eases prostate symptoms, in Germany it is used to treat bladder obstructions – A. INTERESTING NOTE: has been compared to Finasteride for performance. Do NOT take if pregnant or taking hormone therapy. Can cause headache, raised blood pressure, constipation, diarrhea, itching, but in rare cases can cause impotence, or decreased sexual drive. It can take 1-2 months to see results from this herb.

SCULLCAP (also called hoodwort, quaker bonnet)– entire plant- volatile oil, scutellarin, flavonoid, iridoids, tannin, Glutamine, GABA) – sedative, nervine, anti-spasmodic, anti-convulsive, breast pain, expel childbirth, fever, nerve tonic, exhaustion, insomnia sedative, anti-spasmodic, rabies, hysteria muscle spasms, nervous tension, has been used with Schizophrenia, Fibromyalgia, nervousness, anxiety, brings on period, for diarrhea, kidney problems, alcohol and prescription drug withdrawals, epilepsy -C. excess amounts can include drowsiness, giddiness, confusion and finely convulsions

SHEPHERD'S PURSE – herb – Compounds (flavoniods, polypeptides) urinary track infection, lowers fevers, heart and circulatory problems, mild heart failure, low blood pressure and nervous heart complaints, headache, vomiting blood, blood in the urine, diarrhea, premenstrual problems, long periods, and menstrual cramps, superficial burns, internal and external bleeding (is believed it might be the white fungus that grows on it that really does the work)-D warning: can change thyroid function and can cause kidney stones. Do NOT take if breast feeding or pregnant. Do not take if taking CNS depressants

SLIPPERY ELM (also called red elm, moose elm, Indian elm) – The inter part of the bark- Compound (mucilage)- emollient, astringent, antitussive, food poisoning, anti-inflammatory, gastritis, skin injuries, burns, chapped lips, sooths, sore throat, mouth irritations, pneumonia, lung infections, tape worms, rashes and boils, syphilitic eruptions, GERD, Crones disease, ulcerative colitis, diarrhea, mucus membranes, heartburn, peptic ulcer, itchy skin, smokers cough, boils, minor wounds, eczema, insect bites, acne -A.D. warning if taking any prescription drugs take at least 1 hour after using slippery elm. Do not take if you have gallstones or bile duct obstruction. Bark may be abortifacient (can about fetus).

ST JOHNS WORT (also called tipton weed, goat-weed, amber)–
Flowering tops and pedals are used mostly but all above ground parts -
compound (hypericin has been shown to kill the HIV virus)- anti-anxiety,
anti-retro-viral, anti-inflammatory, anti-viral, sedative, anti-depressant,
anti-bacterial, anti-fungal, PMS, fever blisters, sore muscles, bed
wetting, colds, arthritis, heals open wounds, burns, insect bites, - D.
WARNING Causes Photo-sensitivity if used in large quantities.
INTERESTING NOTE: In the 1970's FDA says because of that it is unsafe.
Although they never back rescinded, they say it is safe if used in limited
quantity and can be used as flavoring. Can also cause sedation,
dizziness, and hypomania.
Drug interactions oral contraceptives, Cyclosporin, Digoxin, general
anstesthesia, Indinivir, nefazadone, paroxetine, sertraline, therophylline,
trazadone, Warfin, Xanax, Elavin, Neoral, Gleevec

TEA TREE – leaves- volatile oil, compounds (Terpinen, ethanol) -
antiseptic, antibacterial, anti-fungal, anti-viral, psoriasis, cleanse
infected wounds, burns, coughs, respiratory infections, surgical incisions,
MERSA, acne, dermatitis, boils, athletes foot, warts, ringworm, toenail
fungus, dandruff, vaginal yeast infection, head lice, periodontal disease.
Herpes virus, gingivitis, reduces plaque in mouth, bad breath- B. allergic
reaction to topical use can cause skin irritation or dermatitis.
THYME – leaves, flowers, aerial parts (above ground) – Volatile oil,
Compound,phenol,Thymol- antiseptic, antispasmodic, expectorant,
antibacterial, antiviral, anti fungal, germicide– tonsillitis, cough
suppressant, colds, flu, reduces puffiness, inflammation, asthma,
Bronchitis, digestive disorders, rheumatism, menstrual complaints,
nerves, lung infections, strengthens respiratory system, expectorant,
melancholy, revives a fainting person, sooths sore muscles, sooth
intestinal upset and epileptic attack- D. WARNING: Do NOT take
essential oil into body, do not take too much tea either use mostly as
gargle or external. Buy only distilled twice essential oil. INTERESTING
NOTE: In WW1 thyme oil was used as a battlefield antiseptic. Thyme is
associated with death in many cultures, used as incense in funeral rites,
and used as a fungicide to rid insects from houses, The ancient
Etruscans and Egyptians used thyme oil in embalming their dead.
Ancient Greeks burned thyme in burial rituals and in their temples. In
1994 tobacco companies list of ingredients include thyme oil.

TURMERIC – underground lateral root called the Rhizome – volatile oil,
compound (curcumin) – anti-inflammatory, Anti-cancer, anti-microbial,
hepato-protective (heals ulcers), gas, liver disorders, toothaches, sores,
protects the liver, arthritis, aides in digestion of fats, In India the extract
is sold as an eye wash for conjunctivitis – A.C gall stone caution

VALERIAN– root Rhizome, essential oil, valerenic acid, benzodiazepines, GAMA, valerenol, and a chemically unstable compound (valepotriates)- anti-spasmodic, pain relief, anti-depressant, anti-convulsive , sedative (sleep aide without sleep hangover feeling), calms nervous stomach, stress reliever, anxiety, sedative, digestion problems, nausea, urinary tract problems, American Indians use it for wounds and cuts, migraine, depresses central nervous system, relaxes smooth muscle tissue (stops spasms)- A. D. Warning considered safe but do NOT give to infants. If pregnant consult your doctor before taking it.

WILLOW – bark-(Another choice for divining rods)– tannins, flavonoids, salicin (similar to aspirin)– antioxidant, analgesic, antiseptic, toothache, rheumatism, osteoarthritis, colds, flu, low Back pain, joint pain, headache pain, arthritis, when chewed it relieves fever and inflammation, B. D. WARNING: Since it is similar to aspirin do not use on small children because of chance of Reyes syndrome. Also skin irritation has been reported if allergic quit use and the symptoms will subside. Do not take if
allergic to aspirin. Willow bark affects blood platelets. NOTE: 100mg willow bark has less stomach upset and less effect on blood platelets than 240mg aspirin.

WINTERGREEN – leaves- essential oil (contains 90% methyl salicylate)- headache, muscle pain, arthritis, colds, sciatica, diuretic, essential oil is similar to aspirin- A, B, C, D, WARNING. Considered safe in small amounts, oil of wintergreen is also considered safe but can cause skin irritation in some. Do not take to much internally. NOTE: wintergreen candies now use a flavoring and not the oil. US calls it an over counter Drug.

WITCH HAZEL – leaves, forked branches (used as divining rods)- compound (Tannins)- astringent, antioxidant, antiseptic, anti- inflammatory, soothing skin conditions, hemorrhoids, cuts, Eczema, varicose veins, irritated mouth or throat, reduce fever, menstrual pain, bleeding gums, sprains, feverish colds and cough, back pain, headache, internal bleeding, diarrhea, used commercially in eye wash, lotions, and cosmetics. A.

YARROW- flowers (can use whole plant for poultice for swollen joints) – Volatile oil, compounds (sesquiterpene, lactones, flavoniods)- blood coagulant, anti-spasmodic, antiseptic, astringent, diarrhea, dysentery, arthritis, diuretic, wounds, digestive disorders, fevers, cuts and burns, toothache, swollen joints, cuts, wounds- A.D. Warning. Do not take internally if pregnant. INTERESTING NOTE: Is said to be used by Achilles (for his wounds) – A.

CHAPTER 3 ~HERBS IN THE WILD ~

These are easy to find and grow in most of the US. Warning though, you should get to know your wild flowers by someone who has seen them growing in the wild, an local herbalist or at lease some forestry ranger and also buy a good state wild flower book that specializes on both pictures and very detailed accounts of how they look and grow. Remember the little differences, it could save your life. Herbs like Yarrow look remarkably like Queen Anne's Lace and "Wild parsley" looks a lot like "fool's parsley". One is medicinal and one could kill you. My suggestion is once you think you have found an herb, get a second opinion. You can't be too careful.

Walk gentle upon the earth. Gather from many plants leaving then in good shape when you have gone. Gather leaves after the plant has flowered so it has enough strength to continue it's own cycle of life. When gathering flowers leave some on each plant so it can continue it's cycle. When you need to harvest bark, go out after a storm and pick up the branches and twigs to use their bark. Don't just slice open a tree trunk. If you need to prune a tree use those branches as well. Always apply some mud or wax to the would left by pruning so the tree doesn't get infested in the injury. When harvesting roots pick flatter ground to avoid erosion. If it is a perennial gather in the fall after it has seeded. Other wise early spring or fall is the best time to harvest roots. Respect our mother earth and she will sustain you, don't and we all die.

If you go looking for herbs you might need a little mosquito repellent. Wear light colored long sleeved shirts and pants. Mosquito's love the smell of smelly socks, shoes and scented deodorant. You could reach for the Deet, but instead I suggest Essential oils, Lemon, eucalyptus and geranium. They also hate it when you plant marigold, ageratum and bee balm so those are good scents to use also and a wonderful addition to detour them in any backyard.

If you don't want to bother with a insect repellent try rubbing a dryer sheet on your bare skin and carry it in your pocket.

MOSQUITO REPELLENT (water based)
15 drops in any combination of any of these six essential oils:
bee balm, lemon eucalyptus, calendula (marigold), geranium, ageratum.
1 teaspoon vodka
In a 2 oz spray bottle put the vodka, essential oil and distilled water to fill, shake well and spray lightly over arms, legs and where ever it is needed. Do not spray directly on face.

NOTE: If using a infusion, decoction, or tincture instead of essential oils check the recipe below this one.

MOSQUITO REPELLENT (oil based or infusion)
15 or more drops in any combination of any of these six essential oils
bee balm, lemon eucalyptus, calendula (marigold), geranium, ageratum.
2 oz carrier oil like sweet almond oil.
In a 2 oz bottle put in the essential oils and carrier oil, shake well and
rub over arms, legs and wherever it is needed. Do not put to close to
eyes.

MOSQUITO REPELLENT (from tinctures)
2 teaspoons total from any of these herbs:
bee balm, lemon eucalyptus, calendula (marigold),geranium, ageratum
Made in a tincture of 1 oz vodka or rubbing alcohol. (see tinctures)
In a 2 oz spray bottle put the 2 teaspoons tincture and distilled water to
fill, shake well and spray lightly over arms, legs and where ever it is
needed. Do NOT spray directly on face.

MOSQUITO REPELLENT (from decoction or tea)
In a 2 oz spray bottle add any of "one or more" of the following herb
made into a decoction/tea: bee balm, lemon eucalyptus, calendula
(marigold), geranium, ageratum. Put it in a spray bottle and spray on
skin avoiding the face and eyes.

~ HERBS IN THE WILD ~

BLACK COHOSH – Native to eastern North America. You will find it in
moist shaded woodlands. Shortly after mid-summer it sends up tall
flower stalks that look like bottle brushes towering above dark green
foliage. At first it has tiny pearl shaped buds that open up to resemble a
soft white bottle brush. Honeybees hate them but beetles and flies love
them. Nicknamed bug-bane, bug-wort and black snakeroot. Roots used
in womens tonic. Plant is 1 1/2 foot tall and with flower can be 7 foot
tall. Leaf base is heart shaped or triangular and on top half of leaf it has
serrated teeth.

BLACK HAW a woodsy shrub found in central north America, has olive
sized blue-black fruits hung in clusters. Use root, bark in herbals, fruit
makes wine, jams, jellies and sauces.

BONESET - grows wild across the US. Use leaves and flowering tops

BURDOCK - found roadside and in woods. You will know this plant by
those annoying burs that attach

themselves to everything. Use the root

CHECKERBERRY -Creeping Wintergreen (teaberry)- Found in the woods and clearing especially in areas with moss and peat is used the same as regular wintergreen and has same medicinal value. Plus you can eat the berries. Remember the once popular Teaberry gum. Use the leaves and berries

CLEAVERS - also known as goose-grass is a wild weed. Use the leaves

ELDER TREES - used in grave yards and at burials to protect loved ones from malevolent spirits at bay. Used in protection. A home to the box elder bug. Found in most of the US but not in the pacific north-west. Home of elderberries. Use ripe berries for jams, tonics and syrups. Use flowers for tea and infusions for coughs and colds, rheumatic aches. Use leaves for bruises, sprains, and wounds. In salves for wounds, and healing skin conditions. Extracts of elder flowers for bronchitis, shorten a colds duration, reduce swelling of mucus membranes, nasal and sinus congestion, allergies. Be careful fruit must be cooked or dried. Note some species are poisonous. Since the box elder bug has destroyed so many trees here you may want to stock up if you have access to a live Elder tree. And try what you can to protect it.

FEVERFEW - grows in clearing, by roadside and in meadows. Use leaf.

GARLIC (Wild)grows in woodlands. Use entire plant.

GERMAN CAMOMILE - Grows along road sides, meadows and abandoned places. When crushed gives off a faint scent of apples. Has same uses as Roman chamomile. Use flowers.

GROUND CHERRY - are found all over near streams, slopes and mountain sides as well as woodlands. The cherry is covered in a husk that looks like a Chinese paper lantern. The fruit when ripe is yellow. Do not eat unless it is yellow as it is only non-poisonous when ripe. Also all other parts of plant is poisonous. Eat Ripe cherries only.

DANDELION - grows in lawns. Leaf and root used to create medicines. Flowers used to deep fry or use in wines. Leaves high in potassium. Use leaves, flower or root depending on it's use.

ECHINACEA - grows wild in woods and roadside. Parts used leaves and root.

EVENING OF PRIMROSE - grows wild in north America in fields, roadside and wastelands. Use seeds.

GOLDENSEAL - grows in the woodlands of north America. Is an erect hairy perennial barely a foot high with 1 forked stem with two leaves and has a flower at the base of the stalk leaves have 5- 9 distinct lobes and irregular teeth in the margins. Use the rhizome. Note: Each piece of a rhizome studded with rootlets and underdeveloped buds can be replanted. Harvest after 4-5 years after planting. Each rhizome can be divided into 4-5 new plants at that time.

HATHORN - a tree found in woods through out the US. Use leaves flowers and fruit.

HORSE CHESTNUT - a tree grows in most of the US. Use the fruit.

HORSETAIL - (a weed) in North America has fern like leaves and grows about 18 inches high, in damp woods and roadsides.

JUNIPER - a tree that grows in woods. Use the berries.

LAVENDER - grows wild in meadows and can be bought as seeds or plants in stores in the spring. Use the flowers.

PLANTAIN – grows in most yards in the US. It's leaves lie low to the ground and are wide and oval shaped. They send out a long shoot of what looks like a small and thin cattail but is green or green and dieing grass hued.

MARSHMELLOW - grows wild by roadside ditches and in woodlands by streams. Likes water. Use root.

MILK THISTLE - grows wild in ditches and clearings, Use seeds from seed pods. Can be eaten as snacks as a source of protein and used in place of flax seeds in recipes.

MULLEIN - grows wild roadside and in lawns across the US. As a child we call played with it because it has soft furry leaves. Use the tender young leaves in spring.

PSYLLIUM - (ispaghula) has narrow slender leaves, grown no more than knee high with tiny white flowers on a stem that turn into glossy seeds with a reddish tint. Grows wild in North America, Platago ovata, has the biggest seeds. Dry two or three day then thrash herb to release seeds from pod. Each plant can produce 15,000 seeds. Every 100g produces 71g of soluble fiber

RED RASPBERRY - plant found by roadsides and in clearing. Use all of plant. Considered a womans tonic and good for pregnancy and delivery. Take from 32 weeks gestation until the end shortens second stage of labor and decreases rate of forceps delivery (if taking 1.2 g of dried leaf 2 times a day).

RHODIOLA - small woodsy plant in the succulent family found in moist rocky ledges and northern slopes in the cooler parts of the US. with thick tuberous roots fleshy interior gives off a yellowish tint and when cut gives of a rose like scent. It's pale green leaves have a blueish film that rubs off between fingers. Harvest roots in autumn.

SAW PALMETTO - a palm tree that grows in the south eastern part of the US. Home of the dreaded palmetto bug (a roach by another name) The fruit can be fed to livestock like the early settlers did. Use the berries. (have been told they taste like rotten cheese and tobacco juice mixed) If ripened on the tree the fruit turns black.

SHEPHERDS PURSE - found in woods and roadside, named for it's pouch shaped seed pods. Use the leaves.

SKULLCAP – found in eastern US as far west as Colorado, in rich woods and moist thickets. Flowers grow off side of stem and are small violet colored almost looking like snap dragon but without the snap. Use entire plant.

SLIPPERY ELM - tree grows in the US. Use the Bark.

STINGLING NETTLE - a weed that grows everywhere. The leaves sting you as you pass by. Use Leaves.

ST. JOHNS WORT - found growing wild along roadways and in some yards. Use all above ground parts especially flowers. Grows about 2 feet tall smooth stems usually have ridges and tiny black spots. Inch long tight hugging leaves have netted veins. If they are held up to the light they have translucent dots. Has 5 pedal yellow flowers, about an inch across and bloom in flat topped clusters. June through August. Pick then. Found all across America.

VALERIAN - grows wild in meadows and clearing near lakes and streams. Leaflets and are lance shaped and without teeth. Flowers are tiny white or pink in a crowded flat topped cluster on top of a thick stem, and smell of vanilla. Leaves at base of plant grow 3-25 Grow 1-4 feet tall with lateral roots called Rhizomes. Use those roots

WILLOW - is a tree and is found all over the US. Use the bark.

WITCH HAZEL - is a shrub use bark and leaves. The forked branches are used as divining rods. Use leaves, bark and stems. Found in dry woodlands, near streams, along the edge of bluffs, and almost always on a slope.

YARROW - grows wild along roadways and in meadows (Careful looks a lot like Queen Anne's lace). Also used in potpourris. Use the Flowers.

CHAPTER 4 CREATING YOUR OWN TINCTURE, TONIC OR LIDIMENT

There are different types of tinctures, Vodka, oil, glycerin, rubbing alcohol, apple cider vinegar and witch hazel. They are divided into two basic types of tinctures, an oil base and an astringent (or alcohol) base. You use dried herb with tinctures because it doesn't add extra water to the mix.

Vodka, glycerin, and Brandy tinctures are to be taken internally. Oil can be used either internally or externally depending on the oil used.

Rubbing alcohol, and witch hazel tinctures are for rubs, lotions, ointments, and liniments, or as an astringent base.

Oil can also be used in salves and are usually made with fresh herbs.

Apple cider vinegar can be used for either ligaments or internally.

Whichever liquid you choose the process is done by the basic recipes for each medium and requires the same amount of time for any herb). As long as the herb you use can be used internally you can use it as an internal tincture. Brandy is used when you are making a tonic.

Tonics are traditionally made with 16 Oz's of brandy, vodka or wine, while a tincture is made usually with vodka and 4 Oz's is used.

Know your herbs before starting this. Some you use the leaf, some the flowers, some the root and some you can use more than one part. If using the herbs I covered in chapter 2 you can check there for which part to use.

After you choose an herb you need to consider how you plan to use it. Are you making a salve, a tonic, or are you using it as a tincture for health? Your answer will dictate which type of tincture you wish to make.

VODKA TINCTURE
Can also use brandy, apple cider vinegar, witch hazel, or rubbing alcohol to make this recipe. This method is used when you are taking a health tincture straight into your body. Doses vary so check with each herb. Usual doses range from Usually 1-15 ml per dose.
1 oz dried herb or root
4-6 oz 100 proof vodka
Cover the herb with vodka (just enough to cover but no more) in a 1 qt mason jar with tight lid. Shake daily and store for 2 to 3 weeks depending on the herb strength you want. Some say to put it in the

sunlight, do that only if it says to. If not put it in a cabinet or on counter. Either works well. After the process time strain and put in a dark colored glass jar and store in a cool dark place like a cabinet. Taken internally. NOTE: you can also use witch hazel, rubbing alcohol but do not take internally. Vodka and glycerin Can be taken internally. Apple cider vinegar can be done either way, internally or externally.

OIL TINCTURE
This method is called enfleurage. It is like the vodka tinctures but with oils you don't have the preservative an alcohol has.
3-4 oz herb or root (divided into 1 oz sets)
4-6 oz carrier oil like Sweet almond oil, E.V. Olive oil, sunflower, Jojoba oil, or glycerin
Fill a jar with the leaves and petals of the herb or herbs you wish to make an oil from. Dried herbs. Next, pour oil over them to cover. Tightly cork or cap the jar and keep in a warm place (out of sunlight) for three days. Shake the bottle each day to thoroughly wet the leaves. On the third day strain the oil, fill the jar with fresh leaves or flowers, and pour the same oil back into the jar. Repeat several times until the oil is heavily saturated with the fragrance. Finally, strain the oil through a filter paper or a piece of cloth and store in a tightly caped bottle. This method is used in making salves or rubs and isn't taken internally.

NOTE: Here is an alternative.

ALTERNATIVE METHOD:
You can use 1 oz of herb and put it in a crock pot or on the stove. Either way the time and heat is the same. On warm for 1 hour, Cool and let sit over night. Then heat on warm (once more) for an hour and allow to cool, strain and bottle. It is faster and takes only 1 oz of herb. This is used in lotions, salves and massage oils. To be used internally If making an oil tincture with this method you need to strain and repeat with fresh herb 1-2 more times using a total of 3 -4 oz of herb in all.

GLYCERIN TINCTURE
This can be done like a vodka tincture (recipe below) or an oil tincture (above). Note this is primarily used for diabetics or those who can't take alcohol.
1 oz herb or root
4-6 oz glycerin
Cover the herb with glycerin (just enough to cover but no more) in a 1 qt mason jar with tight lid. Shake daily and store on counter for 2 weeks. After the process time strain and put in a dark colored glass jar and store in a cool dark place like a cabinet. This can be taken internally. Note: if using glycerin do not add a preservative. It will not keep as long as the other tinctures, about 6
 months.

LINIMENT
6 oz any herb, root or bark used as a muscle rub
16 oz apple cider vinegar
Combine in a 1 qt mason jar for 2-3 weeks and strain. Use as a rub over painful joints, swelling or broken bones.

~ ADDING A PRESERVATIVE ~

In vodka or astringent based tinctures there is no need for an extra preservative. But in oil based there is. As a preservative some add Vitamin E oil while others add a few drops of benzoin tincture to the oils as a preservative. If you use vitamin E oil, it is easily obtainable at a natural food store and most drug stores or vitamin shops. You can also use vitamin A or C although I have never used them.

To use vitamin E as a preservative, add 1/4 to 1/2 teaspoon to a tincture you made from the recipes above above

BENZOIN TINCTURE (a preservative)
To make benzoin tincture, soak one tablespoon powdered benzoin in one-fourth cup good-quality vodka or apple cider vinegar for three weeks. Strain and keep tightly corked in a dark bottle. Benzoin is a preservative but it can have a sticky consistency. To use as a preservative add 5-10 drops to the tinctures you made above.

~ SPECIALLITY TINCTURES ~

ASH TINCTURE OR TONIC
For Dropsy (a substitute for quinine) Also helps with leg cramps
1 oz Ash leaves Chopped up
4 oz vodka (if making a tincture)
16 oz white wine (If making a medicinal Tonic)
Put Ash into a 1 qt mason jar with tight lid. Add either vodka or wine. Shake and let sit 14 days, shaking as you remember. Strain and put into a dark colored glass jar with tight lid if tincture, or in a bottle if tonic.

BILBERRY AND CAT'S CLAW TINCTURE
Used for cancer or cancerous tumors
1/2 oz dried Bilberry leaves (break up by hand)
1/2 oz dried Cats claw inter bark
4 oz vodka or brandy

Grind the bark in a coffee grinder and place in a 1 qt mason jar with tight lid. Add the broken bilberry leaves, vodka or brandy, close lid tightly and shake. Let sit 14 days, strain through cheese cloth, and put liquid in a dark tincture bottles. Take 3-5 ml, 3-4 times a day as a regiment.

BILBERRY AND GINKGO BILOBA TINCTURE
For Alzheimer's and diminished brain function
1/2 oz dried Bilberry leaves
1/2 oz dried ginkgo biloba leaves
4 oz vodka or brandy
Place all the above in a 1 qt mason jar with tight lid. Close lid tightly and shake. Let sit 14 days, strain through cheese cloth, and put liquid in a dark tincture bottles. Take 5 ml, 4 times a day as a regiment.

BLACK HAW- GINGER ROOT TINCTURE
For menstrual cramps
1/2 oz Dried black haw root bark
1/2 oz dried ginger root
4 oz vodka or brandy
Grind the two roots in a coffee grinder and place in a 1 qt mason jar with tight lid. Add vodka or brandy, close lid tightly and shake. Let sit 14 days, strain through cheese cloth, and put liquid in a dark tincture bottles. Take 5 ml (1 teaspoon) every 4-6 hours as needed for menstrual cramps.

CALENDULA TINCTURE
For abscesses, throat infections, heal gastric and duodenal ulcers, and stomach ailments.
1 oz dried calendula leaves
4 oz vodka
Put calendula into a 1 qt mason jar with tight lid. Add enough vodka to cover. Shake and let sit 14 days shaking as you remember. Strain and put into a dark colored glass jar with tight lid

CRAMP BARK TINCTURE
To relax muscles
1 oz dried cramp bark
4 oz vodka
Grind root in a coffee grinder and put in a 1 qt mason jar with vodka. Shake and let sit 2 weeks (14 days). Take 5 ml, 3 times a day directly or diluted in water.

TIME OF THE MONTH TINCTURE
For all the aches and pains accompanied with Menstrual Cramps
1/2 oz dried cramp bark

1/2 oz Valerian root
Grind the cramp bark and Valerian root in a coffee grinder and add to the a 1 qt mason jar with the vodka. Steep for 14 days and strain into a tincture bottle or small jar. To use take 1 teaspoon every 2hours as needed for cramps.

ECHINACEA TINCTURE
To use at first sign of a cold
1 oz Echinacea root
4 oz vodka
Grind root in a coffee grinder and put in a 1 qt mason jar with vodka. Shake and let sit 2 weeks (14 days). Take 1-2 ml, 3 times a day directly or diluted in water.

ECHINACEA TINCTURE #2
To use at first sign of a cold
1 oz Echinacea expressed juice from above ground part of plant
4 oz vodka
To do this put through a noodle press. Use 1/4 the juice as you use vodka. Then in a small mason jar allow to sit 1 week. And use as above.
NOTE: must stabilize the juice in vodka at a 1 to 4 ratio.

GINGER TINCTURE (strong)
4 oz ginger root
8 oz vodka
Put dried ginger root through a coffee grinder. Put in a 1 qt mason jar and add to twice as much Vodka. Allow to sit 14 days. Strain and put in a dark glass tincture bottle. Dose is .25-.5 ml, 3 times a day.
NOTE: a weak tincture is made in a 1 to 5 ratio (1 oz root to 5 oz vodka.
To use this you would take 1.5-3.0 ml, 3 times a day

GINKGO TINCTURE
Used for circulation, especially to brain. Used for Alzheimer's and dementia.
1 oz dried Ginkgo leaves
4-6 oz vodka
Put in a 1 qt mason jar with vodka. Shake and let sit 2 weeks (14 days). Strain and place in a dark glass tincture bottle. Take 3-5 ml, 2 times a day.

HAWHORN TINCTURE

Used for Congestive heart failure (mild) OR Mild Hypertension
1 oz dried berries, leaves, flowers or bark
5 oz vodka vodka and allow to sit
If bark is used grind in a coffee grinder before putting into a 1 qt mason jar with a tight fitting lid. And allow to sit 14 days. Strain and put into a dark tincture glass bottle. To use take 12 ml three times aday

LEMON BALM – PEPPERMINT TINCTURE
For cold sores (herpes virus)
3/4 oz dried lemon balm leaves
1/4 oz dried peppermint leaves
4 oz sweet almond oil
Put all of the above in a 1 qt mason jar, close and let sit 14 days. Strain and put into a dark colored glass. To use simply dab on with a q-tip or make the salve-lip balm in Chapter 13.
NOTE: You can make this tincture with vodka if taking internally.

MEADOWSWEET -WHITE WILLOW BARK TINCTURE
Use for pain
3/4 oz dried meadowsweet flower tops
1/4 oz dried white willow bark
4 oz vodka
Put all of the above in a 1 qt mason jar, close and let sit 14 days. Strain and put into a dark colored glass. Take 1-4 ml as needed.

MENOPAUSE TINCTURE
To be used during menopausal transition
1/2 oz dried black cohosh rhizome (main stem root)
1/2 oz dried shatavari
1/2 oz dried chaste tree fruit
6 oz vodka or brandy
Grind in coffee grinder. Place in a 1 qt mason jar with tight lid. Add the vodka or brandy, cap jar and shake. Let sit 14 days and strain. Put strained liquid in dark tincture bottles. Use 5ml (1 teaspoon)morning and at night.

MULLEIN TINCTURE
For the herpes virus
1 oz dried crushed mullein leaves
4 oz vodka

Put into a 1 pt mason jar and allow to sit for 14 days, strain and put into a tincture jar. Take 20-30 drops in water every three hours.

ORRIS ROOT TINCTURE
This is a great replacement for Musk in perfume recipes.
1 oz orris root bruised or sliced (see note below)
4 oz vodka
Put into a mason jar with a tight lid. Steep 14 days and strain. Place in a tincture jar. NOTE: Orris root is the root from an iris flower. Read about orris root under chapter 2 before beginning.

STINGING NETTLE TINCTURE
For prostate problems, BPH
1 oz dried Stinging nettle rhizome
4 oz vodka
Put root through coffee grinder, put in a 1 qt mason jar and add vodka. Allow to set 14 days, strain and place in a dark colored tincture jar. Use 5 ml a day

STINGING NETTLE TINCTURE
For rheumatism, gout, hay fever, or a nutritive supplement
1 oz dried stinging nettle eaves
4 oz vodka
Put root through coffee grinder, put in a 1 qt mason jar and add vodka. Allow to set 14 days, strain and place in a dark colored tincture jar. Use 2-6 ml, 3 times a day

ST. JOHN'S WORT TINCTURE
Used for any of the ailments St. Johns wort is used for (See chapter 2)
1 oz dried St Johns wort flowers
4 oz vodka (just enough to cover)
Put flowers in a 1 qt mason Jar and add vodka. Tighten lid and shake. Let sit 2-3 weeks, strain and place in dark glass tincture bottles with tincture dropper. Take 2-3 dropper fulls in 1 cup hot water or Lemon balm tea.

THYME TINCTURE
Used as a acne zapper or to take down swelling and heal any sore or cut.
1/2 oz dried Thyme leaves
16 oz witch hazel (Can use rubbing alcohol)

Put dried thyme into a 1 qt mason jar and pour witch hazel over it. Let sit 14 days, strain, and put into a dark colored glass jar. To use simply put some on a cotton ball and put in affected area. Do this before bed and if needed again when you wake.

THYME TINCTURE
Used as an antibiotic In WW1.
1 oz dried Thyme
16 oz vodka, witch hazel or rubbing alcohol.
Put dried thyme into a 1 qt mason jar and pour vodka over it. Let sit 14 days, strain, and put into a dark colored glass jar. To use simply put on affected area or on a bandage that you are putting on an area that requires attention.

VALERIAN TINCTURE
For a restful sleep can be taken nightly
1 oz Valerian dried root
4 oz 100 proof vodka
1n a 1 qt mason jar put the herb and vodka. Shake daily for 14 days, strain and put in a dark colored tincture jars with tight lids. Take 5-10 ml 30 minutes before bed time for a restful sleep.

VALERIAN – HOPS TINCTURE
This double acting formula is used for those who really need sleep.
1 oz dried Valerian root
1 oz dried hops flowers
12 oz 100 proof vodka (if needed to cover add two more oz vodka)
1n a 1-2 qt mason jar put the herbs and vodka. Shake daily for 14 days, strain and put in a dark colored tincture jars with tight lids. Take 5-10 ml 30 minutes before bed time for a restful sleep.

WILLOW LIDIMENT
Used for sunburn, muscle aches, and joint pain
6 oz willow bark
16 oz apple cider vinegar
Grind willow bark in a coffee grinder and put in a 1 qt mason jar with tight fitting lid. Add apple cider vinegar and cover and shake. Let sit 14 days. Strain and put in a dark colored jar in a cool dry place.

NOTE: Here are a few herbs and barks that you should not make into tinctures: Aloe, Slippery elm

RECOMMENDED DOSES for some other tinctures

ASTRAGALUS Tincture 2-4 ml, 3 times a day

CHAMOMILE tincture 3-5 ml, 2-3 times a day

FEVERFEW Tincture 5-20 ml, taken in doses throughout the day (for 6 weeks or longer)

GOLDEN SEAL tincture 2-4 ml, 2-3 times a day

HAWTHORN tincture 5 ml, 2 times daily

HOPS tincture 2 ml, 1-3 times a day

PASSION FLOWER tincture 1-2 ml, 1-3 times daily(make w/ hops and lemon balm)

SKULLCAP Tincture 1-4 ml, 1-3 times a day

SAW PALMETTO tincture 1-2 ml, 3 times a day

CHAPTER 5 "COPY CAT" MEDICINE CHEST ITEMS

Home made salves and copy cat on the market products that you can make at home for much less. You can create your own by simply reading the label of ingredients and realizing they go in order of amount used, simply experiment until you get a working product. Happy creating!

EO = Essential Oil

COPY CAT FOR "HERAL SUPPLEMENT TO CONTROL BLOOD PRESSURE"
Their claim is it "Helps work with body and emotions to reduce Blood pressure without side effects". 2 oz bottle sells for $19.95
5 drops Lavender EO
5 drops Ylang-Ylang EO
3 drops Rose EO
2 oz Carrier oil
Mix together in a small bottle and rub into wrist or behind ears daily. This 2 oz container will give you about 5 months of use.

COPY CAT FOR "OLBA'S INHALANT"
A 0.01 tube sells for $8.95 To make this you can either use salt crystals or a combo of salt and bees wax. I will give you both ways. If you have an old bottle you can simply refill it with the essential oils and allow to sit over night so the oil can be absorbed into the canister inside the inhaler.
Salt method
1 teaspoons Epsom salts
4 drops menthol EO
4 drops peppermint EO
6 drops Eucalyptus EO
4 drops Cajeput EO
Put salt into a small glass vile with tight lid and add essential oils. Shake well and inhale as needed.

SOLID INHALANT
1 teaspoon Epsom salts (crushed)
1/2 teaspoons bees wax
5 drops menthol EO
5 drops peppermint EO
7 drops Eucalyptus EO
5 drops Cajeput EO

Melt bees wax in microwave for 15-30 seconds until melted. Add salt and essential oils. Pour into a small glass vile with tight lid (Could use a lip stick tube) and allow to harden before capping. To use, remove the lid and breathe deeply.

COPY CAT FOR "VERTIGO SUPPORT"
Feeling dizzy or unsteady try this herbal supplement. It helps restore calm and focus while soothing anxiety. Use as often as you wish. 2 0z bottle sells for $19.95 in the store
2 oz Jojoba oil
2/3 teaspoon Lavender EO
1/2 teaspoon peppermint EO
1/2 teaspoon neroli EO
1/4 teaspoon anise EO
Just combine the above in a glass bottle and apply to skin and breath deeply.

COPY CAT FOR "BIO-EAR"
A natural remedy to nourish nerve endings and stimulate blood flow and there by quiet the ringing or buzzing in your ear. A 0.5 oz bottle sells for $19.95. This recipe will make 4 bottles.
1/4 teaspoon Aloe Vera juice (optional)
1/4 oz Ginseng root
2 oz sweet almond oil
Place soaked cotton ball in ears for 2-4 hours. Repeat as needed.

COPY CAT FOR "SHINGLE GEL"
Sooths and heals shingles, stops pain, even the pain of healed shingles which were still painful. Comparable to a product sold for cost $34.95 for a 1.4 oz jar
4 oz Aloe gel
20 drops Peppermint oil
5 drops lavender oil
Mix all together and use as needed.

COPY CAT FOR "NEUROPATHY OIL"
A topical formula to ease nerve pain in as little as a week without harmful side effects. Diabetic friendly. 2 oz bottle sells for $29.95
2 oz Organic sunflower oil
1/2 teaspoon marigold EO
1/2 teaspoon peppermint EO
Mix in a 2 oz glass bottle and massage into feet or hands

COPY CAT FOR "FIBROMYALGIA OIL"

An all natural analgesic that temporarily relieves pain, stiffness and numbness without side effects. A 2 oz dropper bottle sells for $29.95

2 oz carrier oil
6 drops eucalyptus EO
6 drops frankincense EO
5 drops myrrh EO
5 drops geranium EO
6 drops peppermint EO
5 drops lemon EO

Mix essential oils into carrier oil. Place in a glass bottle. A roll on top bottle would make application easier. Blend into skin in effective area.

~ SALVES AND CREAMS ~

COPY CAT FOR "HEEL-SPUR CREAM"

Reduces pain and inflammation, This cream is soothing and slightly cool on your heels. A 2 oz jar sells for 19.95

1 (4 oz) container cocoa butter cream (sold at dollar stores for $1-1.50 not the butter)
15 drops devils claw EO
15 drops arnica EO
15 drops Ginger EO
15 drops menthol EO

Mix well and apply as needed. Sells for $19.95 in stores

COPT CAT FOR "WITCH HAZEL SALVE"

A natural remedy for hemorrhoids, rectal irritations and varicose veins. Sooths and tightens while it reduces inflammation. (a 1 oz jar sells for 18.95)

1 oz bees wax
1 teaspoon witch hazel infused oil
1/2 teaspoon vitamin E
4 drops horse chestnut EO
4 drops arnica EO
4 drops chamomile EO

In the microwave melt the bees wax with the olive oil and witch hazel. Then beat together until fluffy add the essential oils and blend well. Put in a sterile jar makes about 3 oz.

COPY CAT FOR "VARICOSE EASE"
Diminish the pain swelling and appearance of varicose veins. See and feel the difference in 6 weeks is their claim.
4 oz cocoa butter
25 drops Horse chestnut EO
25 drops butcher's broom EO
25 drops gotu kola EO
Melt cocoa butter in microwave in 30 second increments. Then add the essential oil mix and pour into a jar.

COPY CAT FOR "TIGER BALM"
Tiger balm is everyones favorite, from headaches to sore tired muscles this stuff cures it all. A (0.63 oz) jar sells for $8.95 Makes approximately 5.5 oz. Or 11 (1/2 oz) jars
4 oz paraffin wax
1 1/2 oz petroleum jelly
10 ml clove oil EO
2 tablespoons camphor EO
2 tablespoons menthol EO
1 oz cajuput oil
1 oz casisa oil
1 teaspoon peppermint EO
Melt the paraffin wax with the cajuput and casisa oil in a pan over a double boiler. Remove from heat. Add the petroleum jelly mixing well to melt and add the essential oils, mix well and beat until lighter.
OPTION 2 just put into small salve jars with tight lids.

SPECIAL NOTE: On Tiger balm – this product has petroleum jelly as an ingredient. Petroleum jelly is flammable. I refuse to use any petroleum product on my skin so instead I use cocoa butter in place of the petroleum jelly.

CHAPTER 6 ~ OTHER "COPYCAT" PRODUCTS

COPY CAT FOR "TUCKERED AND TATTERED BATH SALTSC

Good for aching feet, hands and body due to arthritis, poor circulation, Raynaud's syndrome, or overuse. It also softens your skin while it relaxes you. A 13 oz package sells for $14.95

3 oz Himalayan salts
3 oz dead sea salts
6 oz Epsom salts
10 drops camphor E.O.
10 drops Juniper E.O.
10 drops Thyme E.O.
10 drops Lavender E.O.
10 drops Spearmint E.O.
2 oz Jojoba oil

Blend the essential oils into the Jojoba oil and set a side. Blend the salts together and add the oil mix shaking it to incorporate the oils. Put into a glass jar with tight lid and shake well twice a day for a week. This insures all the oils mix well. Then use 1 oz in a bath as needed. Makes 13 baths.

COPY CAT FOR "JACKIE KENNEDY'S BATH OIL"

Her secret to silky smooth skin and a clear complexion
1 bottle Sweet Almond oil
Just put a tablespoon or two into your hot bath water and soak.

COPY CAT FOR "TEA TREE FOOT SOAK"

A 6 oz box sells for $12.95 and does 6 treatments. Just put 1 oz in a foot bath. Helps eliminate fungus, bacteria and rejuvenates the feet.

3 oz Epsom salts
3 oz Sea salts
20 drops Tea tree EO
10 drops Peppermint EO

Mix together and put into two jelly jars

COPY CAT FOR "NATURE'S APOTHECARYBAROMA MIST "ENERGY"

Was $6.95 for a 2 oz bottle
4 drops black pepper essential oil
3 drops Juniper E.O.
3 drops lavender E.O.
2 drops thyme E.O.
2 drops rosemary E.O.
1 drop geranium E.O.

1 drop neroli E.O.
1 teaspoon 100 proof Vodka
distilled water to fill a 2 oz bottle
Simply mix in the spray bottle and spray into the air in front of you.
~ COPY CAT LIP BALMS ~

NOTE: Something I found out about lip balm containers. Once the lip balm cools it leaves a hole in the center of the tube. Save back a little to re melt and pour into cooled balm after it is set.

COPY CAT FOR "BURT'S BEES LIP SHIMMER"
1 oz sunflower oil
1 teaspoon Castor oil
1 oz beeswax
1/2 oz carndelila wax
1 teaspoon lanolin
1 oz cocoa butter
1/2 teaspoon vitamin E
6 drops peppermint EO
1/4 oz camauba wax
3 drops rosemary leaf EO
a bit of left over lip stick from the bottom of an empty lip stick container OR one Avon sample lip stick to tint balm
Melt the bees wax, cocoa butter, camauba wax, carndelila wax and lip stick sample until melted. Add everything else and pour into lop balm dispensers or lip salve jars. Cap after it cools.

COPY CAT FOR "HEARTH AND HENERY LIP BALM"
Sooths dry, cracked or sunburn lips
1 oz beeswax
1 tablespoon sunflower seed oil
1/4 teaspoon Vitamin E
Melt beeswax in a microwave for 30 second increments until melted and mix well after each time. Add sunflower oil and vitamin E stir well and pour into lip balm containers. Should make 3.

CHAPTER 7 PERFUMES

Creating a "Designer Perfume" Yourself or Designing your own personal fragrance.

Perfumes are labeled different names according to strength of perfume the ascending order according to strength

Perfume / Parfum = very concentrated = used in drops or roll on

Cologne = usually a spray of medium intensity

Toilette water = light fragrance

Splash = lighter than a toilette in fragrance

In the fragrances below the word "With" is used to tell you there is less of those fragrances in the mix.

The ingredients that come before the word "With" are usually used in equal proportions or in ascending order.

Some of the perfumes below have the following ingredients. None of my personal perfumes require the death or torture of any animal unlike Musk (a musk deer is killed to obtain the secretion),
Ambergris (a sperm whale is usually killed for this),
Civer (a glandular secretion from a civet cat which they get through torture.
Castor oil (although the castor oil used in most recipes is made from seeds but the perfume castor oil is taken from Canadian and Russian beavers like musk is from deer. They are killed to get it) For any of those below that require musk I would use orris root tincture. And let sit a
month before using.

You can create these with either flowers or essential oil. The perfume manufactures use essential oils unless stated like with Joy. You could use all fragrance oils but the real products are made with essential oils. I think the aroma therapy aspect of the oils plays as big a role as the fragrance it's self in creating a mood.

Below are the list of ingredients for each perfume. You can create a personal configuration from them to create a truly personal fragrance.

~ CREATING A PERFUME FROM FLOWERS ~

BASIC RECIPE (3-4 teaspoons)
2 cup flowers
1/2 teaspoon 100 proof vodka (to combine and equalize scent)
4 teaspoons water
Smash flowers to a pulp with rock in a ceramic or glass bowl (Or Mortar
and pestle) until it is mush (15-30 minutes, then add the water and
continue to mash a minute more. Let sit 7 days in a jar with a
tight cap and strain into a bottle and add vodka.

~ CREATING A PERFUME FROM ESSENTIAL OIL OR FRAGRANCE OIL~

BASIC RECIPE
1 tablespoon oil
1/4 tsp vodka or musk oil
10 drops essential oil or fragrance oil
shake daily for 7 days to incorporate scent through the entire oil.

~ CREATING A COLOGNE FROM FLOWERS ~

BASIC RECIPE
1 cup water,
1 cup flowers (Smashed like above)
1/2 tsp 100 proof Vodka
Put flowers and water in a jar, Shake and allow to sit 7 days. Strain and
add vodka. Put into a spray bottle.

~ CREATING A COLOGNE FROM ESSENTIAL OILS ~

BASIC RECIPE (2 OZ)
1.75 oz distilled water
20 drops essential oils
1/2 teaspoon 100 proof vodka (To maintain scent.)
Mix together the essential oils in a cologne bottle and add the vodka and
fill with distilled water.

ANOTHER BASIC FORMULA FOR PERFUME
Note this one requires 1 month to cure
1 3/4 teaspoons any blend of essential oils
3 3/4 teaspoons vodka
18 drops orris root tincture

Mix together in a 1 oz bottle and keep in a perfume bottle. Allow to sit 1 month before using this perfume

~ CREATING A TOILETTE WATER WITH ESSENTIAL OILS ~

BASIC TOILETTE WATER
4 oz distilled water
1/2 teaspoon 100 proof Vodka
20 drops essential oil or 1/2 to 1 teaspoon Perfume recipe above

~ MAKING A SPRITZER ~

BASIC SPRITZER
(for hot summer days or to use as air freshener)
Take 1 teaspoon of whatever perfume or cologne you want and put it into a 6-8 oz spray bottle and add 1/2 teaspoon rubbing alcohol and fill with distilled water.
To use on a hot day try putting it in fridge, that way you get a cool spritz of sweet scent.

~ CREATING A COLOGNE STICK ~

BASIC COLOGNE STICK
Perfect for your purse or a little ones purse. Add less fragrance if you want a light stick.
5 drops perfume, cologne or essential oil
1 tablespoon cocoa butter solid
1 tablespoon beeswax
Melt cocoa butter and beeswax, add the perfume, stir well and put in a push up or lip stick container to harden.
NOTE: For a child try lemon essential, cotton candy fragrance oil, lily of the valley, jasmine, spring breeze fragrance oil, or a light rose fragrance.

~ CREATING A PERFUME SOLID ~

BASIC SOLID PERFUME
Perfect for carrying in your purse of taking in your pocket.
1 teaspoon almond oil
1 tablespoon beeswax
5 drops essential or fragrance oil

Heat almond oil and beeswax until melted add the fragrance oil, stir well put in a small pot or tin and cover when completely cool. Of course if you feel the simpler the better and especial for children or those with sensitive noses.

VANILLA KIDS PERFUME
A single vanilla bean immersed in the oil from recipe for a week then added to the recipe's above in place of the oil or vodka makes a wonderfully delicious scent.
NOTE" Also a handful of flowers, bruised and water added to cover for twenty-four hours in a cool dark place then drain the liquid to make a light floral scent.

~ FAMOUS FRAGRANCES ~

"Muguet" by Cody was one of those made from lily of the valley flowers. American scents

Alexandra (One of Alexandra de Markoff Eau de Cologne's created in the 1970's. Is a a delicate yet exotic scent) Jasmine, rose, Iris and marigold.

Ambush Eau de Toilette (by Dana 1955 but soon disappeared from shelves 7.75 oz $15.) -Lavender, heliotrope, bergamot, with orchid, Jasmine, and oakmoss.

Angel perfume - sandalwood, vanilla, patchouli, with a little citrus, melon, peach and plum

Arpege (debuted in 1927 3.3 oz spray for $99. Slogan "Promise her anything but give her Arpege" A soft sultry scent) – bergamot, rose, jasmine, vanilla, and sandalwood.

Blue Grass Eau de Parfum - (sells for $55.00 for a 5.4 oz spray) Carnation and Jasmine with a touch of balsam

Bellodgia -(created in 1927, $75. for 1.7 oz) - carnation, jasmine, rose, lily of the valley

Carnation Eau de Parfum -(introduced in 1942 by Mary Chess. Sells for $55. for 0.33 oz spray) - Carnation with undertones of clove

Classic Blue Grass de Parfum -(by Elizabeth Arden slogan "As fresh as a Kentucky morning" 3.3 oz for $55. fresh sophistication) Carnation, jasmine, with balsam.

Cody's Legendary Eau de Cologne -(Slogan "the fragrance you fell in love with" 1.8 oz for $19.)

Emeraude (one of my mothers favorite's) - Jasmine, orange blossom, and bergamot

Elizabeth Taylor's Gardenia -($40. for 3.3 oz)– gardenia and lily of the valley with white peony and white orchid

Enigma (One of Alexandra de Markoff Eau de Cologne's created in the 1970's. Bestows a captivating allure with spicy notes) Vetiver, allspice, coriander and bergamot.

Interude (created by Frances Denney in 1962. A 2 oz spray goes for $24.00) Oriental citrus blend, patchouli, myrrh, and musk (for shame interlude)

Jungle Gardenia Eau De Parfum (favorite of Actress Barbra Stanwyck and was created in 1932. It's slogan "fresh as a garden in full bloom" sells for $50. for 0.43 oz) gardenia with Jasmine, lily of the valley

"M" Eau de Parfum (A sensual floral by Mariah Carey sells for $65. for a 3.3 oz spray) Tiare flower, gardenia, amber, and Moroccan incense

Norell (from the House of Norell created in 1968. 1 oz goes for $19.95) oakmoss, amber, musk(for shame norell) , jasmine and rose

Oscar de la Renta's Eau de toilette (created in 1977 and winner of the FiFi award 1 oz spray $45.) ylang-ylang, jasmine, lavender, and sandlewood

Samsara (sandskrit word meaning the cycle of birth and rebirth. It is a woodsy floral scent. 1.9 oz spray costs $99. jasmine, ylang-ylang, sandlewood and vanilla

Sun moon stars (my favorite) -fruit oriental floral, orange blossom, amber, musk (for shame Sun moon stars)

White Shoulders (the original honeysuckle scent debuted in Paris in 1932 Eau de Cologne 2.75 oz for $55 slogan "Pamper yourself with White Shoulders) Honey suckle ?

Bal a Versilles (by Jean Desprez in 1961) - Italian bergamot, Italian lemon, neroli, in a base of jasmine and rose, with undertones of sandalwood, vanilla, and vetiver.

Cabochard Eau de Toilette (means headstrong, was created by Madame Gres. She also created many gowns for actresses like Marlene Dietrich. A 3.4 oz spray goes for $49) A base of Vetiver and musk (for shame) then add rose and jasmine.

Femme (by Rochas, created in 1944 in France and favored by Audrey Hepburn a mossy woody scent $89. for 3.3 oz spray) – Vanilla, oak moss and patchouli

Fleurs de Rocaille (created in 1933, $75. for 1.7 oz spray slogan "a memory in every bottle")- Lily of the valley, rose, violet, lilac, jasmine, sandalwood and musk (for shame Femme)

Joy (created by French perfume designer Jean Patou in 1930 to lift the spirits of the great depression. It takes 10,600 jasmine flowers and 28 dozen May roses to create The costliest perfume in the world $99 for 1 oz) Rose with a touch of Jasmine

Lavender Eau de Cologne (from Provence, France, $30. for 6.8 oz) – Lavender essential oil

L' Air Du Temps (By Nina Ricci made in 1948 was a sampling of the flowers so loved in that time. Carnation, gardenia, with an under current of rose, jasmine, iris and sandalwood.

The L'eau des Collines Collection (Perfume of the hills) from Provence, France. Each is 1.7 oz and cost $30.)
Violet - Violet, iris and wild rose
Provence – Lavender, Jasmine and sandalwood
Lavender – Lavender, lemon, patchouli, and musk
Orange Blossom – orange blossom, bergamot and rose

Ma Griffe Eau De Toilette (made in 1940)- Jasmine, neroli, oak moss and musk. (For shame)

Nina Ricci's L'Air du temps (1948 world wide fragrance By French designer Nina Ricci 1.7 oz spray $79.)- Carnation, gardenia, with rose, jasmine, sandalwood and iris

Quelques Fleurs (another favorite of Elizabeth Taylor's) created in 1912 by the "French House of Houbigant" and is still made in Grasse, France. Makes the absolute from 15,000 flowers. But you can make this by simply buying the absolutes ready made. A 1 oz spray bottle goes for $149.00 rose absolute, violet absolute, and jasmine absolute

Sharlimar (Created by French perfumer Guerlain in 1925 The name means "abode of love" as was a tribute to the eternal romance between an Indian Emperor and his wife 2.5 oz spray for $99.) -Vanilla, jasmine, rose, plus other florals they will not tell.

Violet Eau de Cologne (from Provence, France, $30. for 6.8 oz) – violet with a hint of wild rose, and iris

Bluebell (Princess Diana's signature scent by Penhaligon's of London created in 1978, $149. for 1.69 oz spray) citrus, hyacinth, rose, lily, and Jasmine with clove, and cinnamon

Yardley's English lavender ($45. 4.2 oz spray)- Lavender

Yardley's English lily of the valley ($45. 4.2 oz spray) -lily of the valley

Yardley's English Rose ($45. 4.2 oz spray) – Rose

Alvarez Gomez Eau de Cologne (Agua de Colonia Concentratda a fresh citrus masculine scent by Spain's most prestigious perfumer for over 100 years Blending pure plant based oils Name means "Water cologne concentrate" a 3.4 oz splash goes for $40.a fresh citrus scent with a masculine twist) - lemon, eucalyptus, and lavender.

Drakkar Noir Cologne for men -Lavender, sandalwood, spice berries, citrus

Jade East (was made in both cologne and after shave) – bergamot, orange blossom, anise, lemon with notes of oakmoss, sandalwood, and a touch of musk (for shame)

Pino Silvestre (Sells for $34. for 4.2 oz spray and has been around since 1955. It is a woodsy fragrance) Musk (for shame), cedar wood, amber, sandalwood, with oakmoss, patchouli, bergamot and 4 other woodsy fragrances (they aren't telling)

No.4711 (Cologne or aftershave) slogan "Discerning men and women prefer No.4711" 200 year old fragrance) citrus, rosemary and they won't tell.

Royall Cologne's
Lyme (tangy and zesty) lime, clove, nutmeg and pepper
Rugby (masculine scent) pine, geranium and black currant
Spyce is a blend of cloves, cinnamon, nutmeg and pepper.

My personal favorite Perfume blends
Orange blossom and Lime

Jasmine and lily of the valley

Lilly of the valley, Violet and orris root

Rose with vanilla bean

Orange blossom and vanilla bean

Chapter 8 Herbal oils

Remember these need time to draw out the ingredients. Also remember to label and date each thing with both the starting date and date to strain.

Remember "NOT" all oils can be taken internally and oil products are not designed for use internally. The ones that are are Vodka, brandy, or glycerin based.

Warning: Eucalyptus oil if swallowed (even a very small amount) can cause muscle weakness, vomiting, nausea, breathing problems, increased heart rate, and may interact with prescription drugs so consult Doctor right away if swallowed.

CAYENNE MINT SALVE OR OIL
Used when both pain relief and heat is needed
1 cayenne pepper cut and diced
1/4 cup fresh mint
1/2 cup olive oil
Put in a container and shake, leave for 5 days.
This can be made into a salve by adding
4 oz cocoa butter (Melted)
2 oz bees wax. (Melted)
Mix the two melted items into the infused oil and put into salve jars.
Makes 5 (2 oz) jars. To use rub into sore and achy joints or muscles.

CAYENNE DEVIL'S CLAW SALVE OR OIL
Used when both pain relief and heat is needed
1 teaspoon cayenne pepper (from kitchen cabinet)
25 drops Devils claw EO (devils claw is in almost all arthritis over the counter preparations
1/2 cup olive oil
Put in a container and shake. This can be used like this or continue and make it a salve.
This can be made into a salve by adding
4 oz cocoa butter (Melted)
2 oz bees wax. (Melted)
Mix the two melted cocoa butter and beeswax into the infused oil and put into salve jars. Makes 5 (2 oz) jars. To use rub into sore and achy joints or muscles.

HEADACHE MASSAGE OIL

Just dip your fingers into this solution and slowly massage into temples, back of neck and anywhere it hurts.
1 oz carrier oil (almond oil is my favorite for this)
9 drops wintergreen or peppermint E.O.
6 drops lavender E.O.
3 drops Lemon E.O.
1 tab Vitamin E (400 IU)
In a 1 oz vial add the Essential oils and the inside of 1 Vitamin E tab then fill with Almond oil. Shake well and dip your fingers into the oil and massage away your painful headache.

LEMON BALM HEADACHE OIL
A rub for headaches
1 oz lemon balm
1 oz Valerian
12 oz olive oil or sweet almond oil
Allow to sit for 2-3 weeks in sunlight, then strain and use as a headache rub to affected areas

MULLEIN OIL
Relieves earache
1 oz Yellow mullein flowers
enough sweet olive oil to cover
Allow it sit in sun 2-3 weeks and shake daily. Strain and place in a dark glass jar. To use put a 3-4 drops in affected ear. NOTE: do not use if child has ear tubes or drainage from ears.

ST. JOHN'S WORT OIL
For aching joints and back pain
In a 1 qt mason Jar put flowers as they come into bloom. Cover with enough E.O. Olive oil to cover completely. Shake and place in sun for 2-3 weeks. Strain and put in dark colored glass containers. Will Keep 1 year.
To use simply massage into aching joints or back.

THYME OIL
(WW1 Recipe) Used as an antibiotic on wounds
1 oz of herb
12 oz olive oil
Put in a glass jar and cover and let sit in sunlight for 2 weeks shaking it daily. Strain and put into dark vials with tight lids, keep in a cool dark place.

WITCH HAZEL INFUSED OIL

Used in ointments and salves that require an antiseptic, astringent, or pain relieving product.

1/2 oz witch hazel (leaves, bark and or twigs)

6 oz EV. Olive oil

Put in a 1 qt mason jar and shake. Leave 14 days and strain. Put in a dark colored glass jar.

CHAPTER 9 HERBAL TEAS AND INFUSIONS

Teas can be made in bulk and put into resealable single serving and pot size teabags. They make a great present, and handy to have around. You can buy the teabags on line in bulk for very little. To close them up you simply iron shut. Remember to add only the percentages used in each tea mix. To find the best prices on-line use the search terms "Bulk resealable tea bags". If you do not grow the herbs yourself the best way to buy on line is enter the search terms "Bulk herbs". If you are growing them remember to dry them first.

ANISE TEA
Aide digestion, relieves gas, increases milk flow in nursing mothers
1/2 -1 teaspoon anise seeds (crushed)
1 cup boiling water
Crush and steep seeds in boiling water and drink

BASIL TEA
To reduce fevers
2/3 teaspoon dried basil leaves
1/3 teaspoon ground peppercorns
1 cup water
Steep 10 minutes, covering the cup to maintain the volatile oils and drink

BILBERRY (BLUEBERRY) TEA
For diarrhea
1 tablespoon dried berries
2 cups boiling water
Simmer for twenty minutes, Strain. Drink 1/2 cup every 3-4 hours

BLACK HAW TEA
For menstrual cramps, prevent miscarriage, and calms uterine spasms after birth, muscle spasms, small pox, fever, regulate menstrual flow, uterine prolapse, morning sickness, heaving menstrual bleeding, asthma, lowering blood pressure, digestive and urinary cramping, Used by mid-wives following a birth or to prevent miscarriage
2 teaspoons dried root, stem or bark
1 cup boiling water

Steep for 5-7 minutes and drink 1/4 cup every 2-3 hours, No more than two cups daily. NOTE if taking a tincture use 5 ml to 10 ml three times a day

BUTTERWORT TEA
Used for catarrh conditions, asthma, flu, or diseases where there is retention of urine or liquids.
4 teaspoons Butterwort leaves
1 quart of hot water.
Allow to marinate for 5 minutes and take 3 cups daily.

CALENDULA TEA
For ulcers (stomach or throat), throat infections, gum inflammation, gingivitis, after radiation treatments.
1-2 flower head (center flower ring, with or without the pedals)
1 cup boiling water
Steep 10 minutes, strain and drink or use as gargle.

CAT'S CLAW TEA
For asthma, cancer, AIDS, a powerful immune system stimulator, rheumatoid arthritis, HIV, Fibromyalgia, chronic fatigue, shingles, mononucleosis, osteoarthritis, ulcers, neuralgia, gastritis, urinary track infections, kidney problems, fevers, intestinal ailments
1 teaspoon cats claw root/bark
4 cups boiling water
Stir well and pour into a sauce pan and simmer for 10-15 minutes. Cool, strain and drink 1 cup three times a day.

CATNIP TEA
Sleep aide and for menstrual pain
1 teaspoon dried catnip leaves
1 cup boiling water
Steep 10 minutes covering the cup to maintain volatile oils and drink or use as a compress to relieve headaches.

CHAMOMILE TEA
Sleep aide and mild sedative
1 teaspoon chamomile flowers
1 cup boiling water
Steep covered for 15 minutes to receive the most from this brew.

DIARRHEA TEA
If you are out camping and need a cure try this. Also great as a home remedy.
2 teaspoons blackberry or raspberry leaves
1 cup boiling water

Steep leaves in water 10 minutes. Strain or fish out leaves. Drink up to three cups a day. Drink other liquids as well as it is quite astringent.

ENERGY TEA
When you need a lift try this instead of the deadly monster drinks
1/2 teaspoon dried rosemary leaves
1/2 teaspoon dried ginseng root
honey (optional)
1 cup boiling water
Steep ten minutes and drink as wanted for a pick me up

FENNEL TEA
Relieves gas, is an expectorant, sooths coughs, relieves colic (but mix with as much regular water for infants, increases milk production, relieves menstrual cramps.
1/2 teaspoon fennel seeds
1 cup boiling water
Steep ten minutes and strain. Drink

FEVER TEA (gift in a jar)
Makes 3 1/2 cups of mix to either place in a qt mason jar or into individual seal-able teabags. This tea is break a fever In a bowl mix place.
3/4 cup Linden flower
3/4 cup chamomile
3/4 cup spearmint leaves
3/4 cup elder flowers
3/4 cup yarrow
Either place the mixed herbs in a wide mouthed quart jar and add directions or
*Place in 3 teaspoons mix in each regular seal-able teabag or 2 tablespoons in a pot sized seal-able teabag. Write directions on container you keep them in.
**To serve place 3 teaspoons in a large cup of boiling water and allow to steep 10-15 minutes, strain
 and drink
**To serve in a pot place 1 pot sized teabag in a teapot of boiling water and allow to steep 10-15
 minutes and drink
*To serve in a cup place 1 regular sized teabag in a large cup of boiling water and allow to steep 10-
15 minutes and drink.

GINKGO TEA
Good for studying, tests, and used in a dementia or Alzheimer regiment
1 teaspoon dried ginkgo leaves

1 cup boiling water
Steep 10 minutes and drink 3 or more times a day

GOLDENSEAL TEA
It is extremely bitter. Used for mouth sores, canker sores, cracked and bleeding lips. Can be used as a eyewash and will sooth eye allergies (is used in a popular commercial eye drop to do that (Moisten a cloth and wipe eye while closed, or apply 1 drop in each eye (But use the 2 cups to make it for eye wash).
1/2 teaspoon goldenseal root
1-2 cups boiling water
Steep 10-15 minutes and drink or use as a wash

HOPS ANTI-ANXIETY TEA
Also works with catnip
2 teaspoons dried hops
1 cup boiling water
Steep 5-7 minutes, strain and drink. Three times a day

HYSSOP TEA
Can be used as a tea or a gargle to relieve cold, coughs, soreness and as an expectorant.
1 teaspoon hyssop herb
1 cup boiling water
Place a cover over while it steeps and steep 10 minutes. Drink or gargle.

JUNIPER TEA
Used for arthritis, stomachache, colds and as a diuretic.
5-10 juniper berries crushed
1 cup boiling water
Steep 10-15 minutes and drink

LEMON BALM TEA
Used to induce perspiration to relieve fever from colds and flu, also menstrual cramps, insomnia, relieves gas and bloating, headache and nerves.
5-6 dried lemon balm leaves
1 cup boiling water
Cover with a top, Steep 7-10 minutes and drink, can add honey and mint if desired

LEMON BALM TEA
Used as a calmative or to relieve headaches.
1/4 oz dried lemon balm leaves
1 cup boiling water

Cover with a top, Steep 7-10 minutes, strain and drink, can add honey if desired, also okay for children although I would lower the dose to 1/2 cup.

MEADOWSWEET TEA
For digestion, dyspepsia, ulceration, rheumatic pain, diarrhea (even in children).
1/6 oz dried flower tops
1 cup boiling water
Allow to steep 5-7 minutes, strain and drink 3 times a day.

MIGRAINE TEA
Need I say more, TRY IT.
2 1/2 cups water
3 teaspoons dried ladies mantle leaves
3 teaspoons dried peppermint leaves
Bring to a boil all ingredients and boil lightly 20 minutes. Remove from heat and steep covered another 10 minutes. Strain into a cup and sip slowly in a dark quite room.

MARSHMALLOW ROOT TEA
Relieves sore throat, coughs, bronchitis, urinary track infections, colitis, eases constipation, sooths inflamed throat tissues.
1 teaspoon sliced or grated marshmallow root
1 cup boiling water
Steep 10-15 minutes and drink

MULLEIN TEA
For Herpes virus
2 heaping tsp of dried mullein flowers and leaves
1 cup boiling water.
Steep 10 minutes and drink 6-8 cups a day for herpes viruses. Can also be applied to effected area to sooth.

PEPPERMINT TEA
Relieves stomach aches or bronchial conditions
1-2 teaspoons peppermint leaves or (3 drops peppermint essential oil)
1 cup boiling water
Steep if using leaves (10 minutes)strain and drink. If you use lemon thyme you will not need any sweetener.

RASPBERRY LEAF TEA
Used as a womans tonic, pregnancy tea and for diarrhea (see notes under wild herbs section)
1-2 teaspoons dried leaves
1 cup boiling water

Steep 5 minutes. Drink 1-2 cups three times a day
NOTE If using as an extract for diarrhea you need to steep 15-30
minutes to extract the tannins.
Then take 1/2 cup three times a day.
Can sweeten it with honey and or lemon.

SLIPPERY ELM TEA
For sore throats, cough, bronchitis, colds and flu
1 Tablespoon slippery elm bark
 (powder)
1 c. water, boiling
1 T. sweetener (honey, raw sugar)
2-3 oz milk
Mix well and drink slowly allowing it to coat your throat.

THYME TEA
Expectorant and coats the back of your throat, also for colds and flu,
menstrual cramps, digestion, lung infections.
1 teaspoon dried thyme leaves (I love lemon thyme for this)
1 cup boiling water
Cover with a saucer to keep volatile oils in. Steep 10 minutes and strain,
add honey to taste.

WILLOW BARK TEA
For pain and inflammation
1 teaspoon willow bark
1 cup boiling water
Steep 10 minutes, strain and drink.

WINTERGREEN TEA
Used to treat arthritis pain, headache, cold symptoms and sore muscles.
Note: take only 1-2 cups a day.
1 teaspoon fresh wintergreen leaves crushed
1 cup boiling water
Bruise leaves and steep 10 minutes. Drink.

~ SPECIALTY BLENDS ~
Made to either fill a pot, or make in bulk make into tea bags.

NIGHTY NIGHT TEA (Makes a teapot full)
For a blissful sleep
1 tablespoon lemon balm leaves
1 teaspoon skullcap leaves
1 teaspoon passion flower leaves

1/2 teaspoon chopped Valerian root
Place in a teapot with 2 cups boiling water. Steep 10 minutes, strain and drink. Sweeten with honey if
wanted.

CLARI-TEA
Great for reviving from afternoon slump.
1 oz dried ginkgo leaves
1 oz green tea
Mix together and put into resealable tea bags or keep in a glass jar with a tight fitting lid.
TO USE:
1 heaping teaspoon herb mix
1 cup boiling water
steep 5-7 minutes, strain and drink.

COLD TEA
A cold care system in one tea
2 oz Echinacea root
1 oz each hyssop, thyme and peppermint leaf
Use 1 tablespoon in 1 cup boiling water, steep 15 minutes, strain and drink. Drink three cups a day.

COLD- HOARSENESS TEA
To sooth your throat
2 oz Malva flowers
1 1/2 oz Mullein flowers
Use 2 tbs of mixture per 1 cup hot water. Steep 10 minutes; strain.

ENGLISH ROSE TEA
Enjoy a great cup of medicinal tea
1/2 cup dried Red Rose petals
2 tablespoons dried Lemon Balm
1 tablespoon dried Rosemary
Mix well. Use 1 teaspoon for each cup.

BLADDER INFECTION TEA
The name says it all
1 1/2 oz dried Goldenrod
3/4 oz chopped Dandelion root
3/4 oz chopped Rose Hips
1/4 oz Juniper Berries*
Pour 1 cup boiling water over 2 tsp of mixture. Steep 10 minutes & strain.
NOTE: *can become toxic, so only drink 2 cups of this mixture daily for no more than 3 days

ELDER FLOWER TEA

A mild stimulant and to induce perspiration.

1 oz dried elder flowers
1 oz dried peppermint
1 oz dried Yarrow flowers

To create tea mix equal parts of each and take 1 teaspoon of mix with 1 cup of water and steep 10minutes.

CHAPTER 10 MAKE IT YOURSELF PRODUCTS

THYME MOUTHWASH
Used to treat inflammations of the mouth, toothache and throat infections.
3 drops Thyme oil
3 oz distilled water
Mix together, swish and spit.
If making tooth paste mix the first three together. Then add the flavor and mix again, put in a squeeze tube or a jar and use a Popsicle stick to get out.
If making dry tooth paste omit the glycerin and shake very well, wait a day and shake again. Break up any clumps and shake again. Then put in a small bottle. Shake out some on a wet tooth brush to use.

MINTY MOUTHWASH
 (Makes 6 oz.)
1/4 cup aloe juice (not gel)
1/4 cup witch hazel infusion (see below)
2 oz distilled water
1 drop tea tree E.O.
2 drops Peppermint E.O.
Mix together, swish and spit.

WITCH HAZEL INFUSION
1 teaspoon witch hazel plant material
1 cup boiling water
Steep 10 minutes strain.

WITCH HAZEL ACNE CLEANSER
1 recipe witch hazel infusion (from above)
10 drops peppermint E.O.
Mix together and use with a cotton ball on affected area.
***An alternative is to buy witch hazel solution at beauty counter and add 10 drops peppermint per 8 oz of product. Shake lightly and use.

TOOTH PASTE OR TOOTH POWDER
4 tablespoons baking soda
1 tablespoon salt
2 tablespoons glycerin (FOR PASTE)
3 drops one of the following (Peppermint, cinnamon oil, thyme, or Lemon E.O.)
Mix the baking soda, salt and EO to make a powder. Simply shake well and break up clumps.
For paste add the glycerin to the mix above.

NAIL STREGTHENER

Stops splitting, chipping, peeling, and breaking nails, restores nails to health. To use simply rub into your nail beds.

2 tablespoon Glycerin
1 tablespoon lanolin
1/2 oz bees wax
1 tablespoon wheat germ oil or grape-seed extract
1 cap 400 IU vitamin E

Melt beeswax with wheat germ oil and whisk together or stir in the rest. Put into a small jar with a tight lid.

HIVE LOTION

Great for food allergies or emotional hives

2 oz distilled water
1 tablet Vitamin E (400 IU)(Prick and use the liquid inside)
20 drops lavender E.O.

In a 2 oz glass bottle with a tight lid put in the Vitamin E and the essential oil then add the distilled water. Shake well and dab on hives with a cotton ball.

ANTIBACTERIAL OIL

This is great for boils but can be used on cuts and scrapes also.

1 oz carrier oil
25 drops tea tree E.O.
25 drops lavender E.O.
15 drops thyme E.O.

To use for boils- first apply a hot compress for 10 minutes. After you take it off apply this oil and cover loosely with a dressing. Repeat every two hours.

**For cuts and scrapes- simply wash cut and apply this oil. Cover with bandage if you wish.

RINGWORM PLASTER

With some mustard seed and a little thyme or sage from your spice rack you save yourself a bill from a dermatologist.

1 tablespoon Mustard seed
1 teaspoon thyme or sage
a few drops apple cider vinegar

Pulverize the seeds and leaves with a motor and pestle and place it in a small bowl. Add a few drops apple cider vinegar and mix to create a paste. Then apply to the affected area and cover with a bandage. Reapply once a day until gone.

SLEEP LOTION

A great lotion for kids that are away from home, people with to much to think about and elderly who just can't sleep.

1 oz unscented lotion
10 drops lavender EO

Mix together and put in a 1 oz pump bottle.

To use pump a small dot onto wrist, rub wrists together and lay with wrists near your nose, breath deeply.

WART REMOVER

For this one you will have to go out into your yard. Freshly picked dandelion stalks. Apply the milky liquid onto your wart being careful not to touch your skin beside the wart. Do this 2 times a day for several days until the wart lifts from the skin. You can apply a bandage if you wish

during this process so as to not smear it onto sensitive skin. This can be done with kids as well. Keep liquid out of eyes.

~SPRAYS ~

SLEEPY TIME BEDDING SPRAY

For a restful sleep
2 oz distilled water to fill
20 drops lavender E.O
1/8 teaspoon vodka

Put in a 1 oz spray bottle and spray pillow before going to bed.

ECHINACEA SAGE SPRAY

For sore throats and coughs
1/2 teaspoon Echinacea
1/2 teaspoon sage

In 1/2 cup boiling water, steep 10-15 minutes and pour into a spray bottle. Spray sore throat as needed.

ANTISEPTIC SPRAY (better than the standard, Phenol)

2 oz sweet almond oil
8 drops sweet orange oil
5 drops lavender
5 drops lemon-grass

Put into a 2 oz spray bottle and use on cuts, scrapes, or infections.

LEMON HAIR SPRAY
1 cup distilled water
5 drops lemon EO
1 tablespoon aloe juice
Mix all together in a spray bottle and shake well before spraying on hair.

~ SYRUPS ~

BILBERRY SYRUP (blueberry)
Eyes health, antioxidant, protects from heart disease, preserves brain function, inflammation, and helps with any degeneration disease.
1 1/2 cups fresh or frozen bilberries (blueberries)
1 tablespoon lemon juice
2 tablespoons dark honey
pinch of ground cloves
Add ¼ cup water if using fresh berries.
Bring to a boil, reduce heat and simmer 10 minutes. Refrigerate or can in boiling water bath for 10 minutes.
To use:
*2 tablespoons in sparkling water creates a wonderful drink.
**2 tablespoons in a yogurt smoothie,
***2 tablespoons in 1/2 cup olive oil and one clove minced garlic for a salad dressing.
****Serve over pancakes, in milk, or over ice cream. You can even add to ice cream while making it before you freeze it.

BUTTERWORT SYRUP
2 lbs bruised leaves
Placed in 5 pints of boiling water and left 24 hours (covered). Strain and measure in as much sugar as infused water. Bring to a boil and reduce heat and continue a low boil until it becomes syrupy. At that point you can either place cooled in the fridge or process in boiling water baths for a canned product.

CHERRY COUGH SYRUP
Great tasting, well working cough syrup even the kids will take.
2 cups of cherries
A few lemon slices
2 cups of honey

Place cherries in a pan and add just enough water to cover. Add lemon slices and honey. Simmer the mixture until cherries are soft. Remove from heat. Remove the lemon slices and the cherry pits from the mixture. Refrigerate and take several tablespoons as needed for coughing.

Wild cherry bark cough syrup
Cover the bottom of a crock pot with Wild Cherry Bark Cover entirely with honey. (can also be done with Violet leaves and flowers).
Set on warm heat for two days and stir occasionally.

ELDERBERRY SYRUP
For influenza. It shortens the time by 3-4 days.
2 pounds rinsed elderberries
4 cups water
Place in a sauce pan. Bring to a boil and simmer 20 minutes. Strain cooled mix and discard the seeds after pressing out all the juice, stir in 2 1/2 cups sugar and cook over medium heat until it becomes a syrup. Can in boiling water bath 10 minutes or place in fridge. Wonderful over pancakes, sponge cake, added to a shake, over ice cream, or put in milk. Or simply take 1-2 tablespoons at the onset of influenza.

ELDERBERRY COLD AND SORE-THROAT SYRUP
2 1/2 cups ripe elderberries
1/2 cup sugar
1 cup water
Boil gently until the constancy of a thick sugar syrup. Take 1 1/2 – 2 oz to get rid of a chill or as a gargle for sore throat.

ELDER FLOWER VINEGAR
You can use as part of a dressing recipe for salads, to marinate vegetables, as an elixir either plain or in water.
1/2 cup elder flowers
6 cups apple cider vinegar
Steep for 12-14 days strain.
*As a elixir take 15 ml three times a day at the first sign of cold symptoms

FENNEL COUGH SYRUP
For coughs
2 teaspoons fennel seeds
3 tablespoons honey

1 cup water
In a small sauce pan place the seeds, honey and water and bring to a boil. Simmer on low 20 minutes. Remove from heat and strain. Store in fridge for up to a week.
To use take 1 tablespoon every 3-4 hours as needed for a cough or cold.

HATHORN SYRUP
As part of a heart healthy diet use on pancakes.
1 cup fresh hawthorn berries or 1/2 cup dried berries
3 cups water
In a sauce pan simmer 10 minutes, mash and simmer 10 more minutes, strain and put liquid back in pan with 1 cup honey. Simmer until it dissolves and store in fridge up to three weeks or can in a boiling water bath 10-15 minutes.

HOREHOUND COUGH DROPS
These are a little harder to make than the pastilles but so worth the work. Need a candy thermometer.
2 oz dried horehound leaves
3 1/2 cups dark brown sugar
20 drops eucalyptus E.O.
10 drops wintergreen E.O.
20 drops Tea tree E.O.
3 cups boiling water
In a heat proof container pour boiling water over dried horehound leaves and steep 30 minutes over low heat and strain. In a pan heat liquid to boil with brown sugar. Continue boiling until it reaches 295 degrees on a candy thermometer take off heat, stir in essential oils and let cool slightly and with buttered hands roll into small balls smash slightly and set on waxed paper to dry and harden completely. Wrap individually in plastic wrap

KITCHEN CABNET COUGH SUPPRESSANT
1/4 teaspoon ground cayenne pepper
1/4 teaspoon ground ginger
1 tablespoon apple cider vinegar
2 teaspoons water
2 tablespoons honey
Dissolve the cayenne and ginger in vinegar and water. Add the honey and mix well. Take 1 tablespoon as needed for cough. Keep in a tight lidded small container.

MARSHMELLOW ROOT COUGH SYRUP
For coughs
2 cups water

2 cups sugar
1/4 cup juice from an orange or lemon
1 1/2 to 2 1/2 tsp chopped dried marshmallow root
In a small saucepan, bring the marshmallow root and water to a boil.
Reduce heat to low and simmer for 20 minutes. Strain liquid into
another saucepan. Will give you about 1 cup. Over a low heat, slowly stir
in the sugar until it becomes thick and granules completely dissolve. You
can add more water if the mixture becomes too thick. Remove from
heat, stir
in the orange juice. Transfer to a container and allow to cool before
covering tightly. Use 1 tablespoon as needed.

WILD VIOLET COUGH SYRUP
For coughs.
1/2 cup plus 2 T violet flowers, cleaned
1 quart water
7-1/2 cups sugar
Remove the little white part at the base of the petals. Then steep the
petals in hot water overnight. The next day, filter this infusion and melt
the sugar into it, slowly, until you get a syrupy consistency. Take 4
tablespoons a day for light coughs and sore throats.

SORE THROAT PASTILLES
Sore throat lozenges are easy to make and can travel with you
anywhere.
1/4 cup dried violet pedals
1/4 cup dried rose pedals
1 teaspoon dried marshmallow root
honey
confectioners sugar
With a mortar and pestle crush violet and rose pedals to powder. Then
do the same to the marshmallow root. Mix with honey to form a ball. If
to thick add a little more honey if to thin add some confectioners sugar.
Roll into pea sized balls allow to dry on waxed paper for 48 hours and
wrap in
plastic wrap individually and store in a cool dry place. For sore throat
and light cough

Whooping Cough Syrup
Cough syrup used by grandmother's when their children had bad colds.
It is a very reliable mixture.
1/2 lb flax seed
6 lemons [juice]
1 cup granulated sugar

1/2 pound honey
Put flax seed in bag; pour over it 1 1/2 pints of water. let simmer down to 1/2 the amount; remove from fire and add other ingredients while still hot. dose; give any amount as often as needed. Half of recipe makes enough for 1 pint

~ ELIXIRS AND TONICS ~

BILBERRY CORDIAL (blueberry)
For stomach upset.
2 cups blueberries
3 cups brandy (24 oz)
1 1/2 cups honey
Combine berries with 2 c. brandy, steep for 1 week. strain through jelly bag. Add remaining brandy
 and honey, bottle.
 (The longer you can let this sit, the better.)

CARAWAY CORDIAL(stimulant)
1 oz smashed caraway seeds
6 oz sugar
1 qt brandy
Steep the above for 3 weeks, strain and bottle
CARAWAY CORDIAL (stimulant)
1/2 cup of smashed caraway seeds
2 quarts of vodka
1/2 cup sugar
Mix together and steep for 14 days, strain and bottle

ELDERFLOWER CORDIAL
For cold or flu symptoms.
3/4 pound sugar
1 quart vodka
4 medium lemons
10 large elderflower heads. Shake to remove insects
Place everything in a large mason jar or other glass seal-able container. Allow to sit 14days and strain.

RHODIOLA ELIXIR

For stress, fatigue, depression, anxiety or for stamina, endurance, and CFS
1 oz rhodiola rhizome root
4 oz apricot brandy
1 cinnamon stick
Grind root in coffee grinder and place in a 1 qt mason jar with apricot brandy (or 8 oz vodka and 1 oz dried apricots). Allow to sit 14 days, strain and put in a dark elixir bottle. Take 1 teaspoon, 1-2 times a day as an tonic

~ INFUSIONS AND INHALERS ~

RESPIRATORY INFUSION
2 drops each of eucalyptus EO, Lavender EO, and tea tree EO in a heat proof bowl with
2-3 cups boiling water.
Stick a towel over head and head over bowl, breathe in deeply.
To relieve stress
***Used as an inhalant -
5 drops chamomile E.O.
Put in a handkerchief and breathe in.
**As a spray - put the essential oil in a 1 oz spray bottle with distilled water. Add 1/8 teaspoon vodka to stabilize.

RESPIRATORY INHALER
Fill a small vial with a tight fitting lid with
1/2 oz rock salt
then add
6 drops each of eucalyptus EO, Lavender EO, and Tea Tree EO.
Cap and allow to sit 24 hours before using. To use simply take the cap off and inhale deeply.

INHALER
1/2 oz rock salt
25 drops rosemary EO (or peppermint, spearmint, eucalyptus)
1 bottle
Place the salt and oil in a very small amber or dark blue bottle. Close with a lid and shake. Sniff as needed to clear up your nasal passages.

YET ANOTHER INHALER
1 teaspoon rock salt

8 drops peppermint E.O.
8 drops eucalyptus E.O.
8 drops wintergreen E.O.
Put salt in a small glass vial and add essential oils. Shake well and inhale as needed.

CHAPTER 11 SALVES, OINTMENTS, POULTICES, CREAMS, RUBS, BALMS, AND OTHER INTERESTING STUFF

When making anything herbal, Always remember to label and date any product along with a list of ingredients. That way you know at a glance what is in it. I usually put right on the container what it is used for and how to use it also.

A basic recipe will allow you to create salves using your own herbs that you have grown or use any essential oil to create salves for any use under the sun.

BASIC SALVE
*Number 1 (using infused oil)
4 oz cocoa butter or Shea butter
1-2 oz oil infused (See CHAPTER 8)
1/2 teaspoon vitamin E
Melt cocoa butter, add oil and vitamin E and put into jars to cool then cap, label and date.

**Number 2 (using Essential oil)
4 oz cocoa butter or Shea butter
1/2 teaspoon Vitamin E
1-2 oz oil (almond or olive)
25 drops any Essential oil
Melt cocoa butter and oil together then add vitamin E and put into jars to cool then cap, label and date.

~ AN ASSORTMENT OF RECIPES USING ESSENTIAL OILS ~

ACNE OVERNIGH CREAM
Apply this at night and wash off in the morning
1 tablespoon cosmetic clay (any color or kind)
10 drops tea tree E.O.
A few drops Vitamin E oil
In a small bowl mix the cosmetic clay with the essential oil then add a drop or two Vitamin E to make a good paste. To use simply apply to problem areas at night after washing your face. This fits well in a lip balm jar from many stores sample isle where they have empty containers. I use the yellow one for this.

ACNE

I like witch hazel for this one as both work well on acne giving you double the power.

1 oz distilled water, witch hazel or rubbing alcohol (choose one)
5 drops tea tree EO
2 drops peppermint or lavender essential oil.

Mix and apply with a cotton ball, Keep any leftover in a glass jar with tight lid in the medicine cabinet.

ACNE MUSCLE SALVE

3 oz cocoa butter
1 oz beeswax
7 drops peppermint EO
5 drops Eucalyptus EO
5 drops Thyme EO

Heat cocoa butter and beeswax until melted, add the essential oils and put into 1-2 salve jars. Makes 4 oz total.

BETTER THAN "TIGER BALM" "

Tiger balm is everyones favorite, from headaches to sore tired muscles this stuff cures it all. A 1/2 oz jar sells for $8.95 Makes 10 jars of 1/2 oz or 5 (1 oz) jars.

2 (1 oz) bars bees wax
3 oz cocoa butter
1 oz clove oil EO
1 oz camphor EO
1 tablespoon peppermint EO
1 teaspoon cinnamon EO
1 oz eucalyptus EO

Melt the beeswax and add the essential oils, mix well and put into small salve jars.

COLD AND FLU SALVE

To use you can put on your chest, under your nose, or on the bottom of your feet like with the popular store bought chest rub.

1 oz beeswax
2 oz cocoa butter
1 oz coconut oil
10 drops eucalyptus EO
5 drops camphor EO
5 drops Peppermint EO

5 drops tea tree EO
Heat beeswax, cocoa butter and coconut oil until melted then add the Essential oils and stir well. Put into a salve jar. Makes 4 oz

CUTICLE CREAM
Need I say more
1 tablespoon bees wax
1 tablespoon cocoa butter
5 drops lemon essential oil
1 teaspoon Vitamin E
Melt cocoa butter and bees wax add the rest and stir well. Put in a salve container. Makes about 0.5
 oz

DECONGESTANT SALVE
Makes 5 oz and works wonderfully
4 oz Sweet almond oil
1/2 oz peppermint E.O. (2 tablespoons)
1/2 oz eucalyptus E.O. (2 tablespoons)
1/2 oz wintergreen E.O. (2 tablespoons)
4 drops tincture of benzoin
1 oz grated beeswax
Add oil and beeswax together and melt in microwave or stove top. Stir in the essential oils and tincture. Pour into a clean wide mouth Jar or two with tight lids. Allow to cool before capping. Put on chest, under nose, inhale from jar or place on bottom of feet at night and cover with cotton socks while you sleep.
NOTE: Can make it into a roll-on either in a reusable deodorant screw up container or in a lip stick roll up container for easy applications.

HEADACHE RELIEF SALVE
2 oz beeswax
3 oz cocoa butter or Shea butter
3 oz sweet almond oil or olive oil
25 drops lavender EO.
Melt beeswax and cocoa butter until melted. Add oil and warm a minute. Then add the essential oil and pour into 8 (1 oz jars)

HOT PEPPER RUB
The Capsaicin in hot peppers is used in many drug store remedies
2 tablespoons ground cayenne pepper
1/2 cup aloe vera gel
1/2 teaspoon vitamin E
1/2 oz beeswax

1/4 cup almond oil
In almond oil place the cayenne pepper,allow to sit over night. Melt bees wax with cayenne and oil. Then take off heat With a hand beater add the vitamin E and aloe beating until well blended. Place in a 8 oz jar with tight lid (or 2 (4oz) jars).

SPORTS RUB
For sore muscles
1 oz carrier oil add EO
3 drops rosemary EO
2 drops lavender EO
1 drop eucalyptus EO
Blend together in a flip top bottle and rub onto joints before doing strenuous exercises or running.

PAIN- HEALING SALVE
Relieves pain from arthritis and over used muscles and heals cuts and scrapes.
1 oz cocoa butter
1/2 oz coconut oil
5 drops grape seed essential oil
10 drops devils claw essential oil
5 drops peppermint essential oil
5 drops lavender essential oil
Heat cocoa butter and coconut oil until melted then add the rest and mix well. Place in a salve jar. Makes 1.5 oz

PEPPERMINT LOTION BARS
These bars are great for cracked feet or skin. The peppermint is both soothing and healing.
4 oz beeswax
4 oz coconut oil
4 oz sweet almond oil
1 teaspoon Peppermint E.O.
2 oz cocoa butter
Melt bees wax, coconut oil, cocoa butter and sweet oil in Microwave in 30 second cycles until melted. Mix in peppermint Essential oil and then pour into a push up dispenser (Like an old deodorant container) or a soap mold. I use a valentine heart mold.

STIFF OR SORE COMPRESS
For either swollen glands. or Stiff neck
5 drops Lavender essential oil

5 drops bergamot essential oil
2 drop Tea Tree essential oil
2 Cups hot water
Mix together. While still warm, soak a soft flannel cloth in the water and wring it out. Wrap it around the neck. Cover with a towel to hold in the heat. Remove before it becomes cold. Repeat as desired.

PAINFUL JOINTS LINIMENT
A wonderful blend
8 teaspoons Castor oil
4 tablespoons glycerin
4 tablespoons Aloe Vera gel
4 tablespoons cayenne tincture
1 teaspoon Vitamin E
40 drops wintergreen E.O. (1 2/3 teaspoon)
Put in a 4 oz small glass jar with tight lid and shake. Massage over sore joints.

ACNE CLEANSING PADS
This is wonderful for the teenager in the house or anyone with an acne problem
1 1/2 cups distilled water
1 tablespoon dried yarrow
1 tablespoon dried Chamomile
12 drops tincture of benzoin
5 drops Wintergreen E.O or Peppermint E.O.
Cotton Cosmetic pads
In a pan heat water and herbs to boiling and boil 2 minutes. Take off heat and cover for 30 minutes. Strain and add the essential oil and tincture. Mix well and place in a open mouthed glass jar. (the salsa jar you find in the chip isle is perfect. It is a glass jar) Add the cosmetic pads and fill with water. This will make 2 jars, one for a friend.

HEMORRHOID PADS
Make these at home for a fraction of the cost. Wonderful for anyone who suffers from them.
1 oz witch hazel (recipe in this book or store bought)
5 drops cypress E.O.
3 drops geranium E.O.
5 drops lavender E.O.
2 tablespoons Aloe Vera gel (from plant or store bought)
cotton cosmetic pads (not cotton balls)

In an open mouthed jar with tight lid mix all the ingredients until well blended. Add the pads to saturate. Put in the fridge for an hour or more and apply to inflamed area as needed.

DECONGESTANT
For humidifiers or on top of wood burners (in winter).
On a cotton ball place
4 drops wintergreen E.O.
4 drops peppermint E.O.
4 drops eucalyptus E.O.
For a humidifier place near the vent to disperse. If on a wood burner either float the cotton ball on milk cap in a heat proof container like a pan filled with water or simply place the cotton ball into the water and place on the wood-burner. (of course the wood burner has to be lit)
~ MORE RECIPES USING HERBS ~

ARNICA BALM
Used for bruising
1 oz arnica leaf
4 oz almond oil
3 oz beeswax
1 teaspoon Vitamin E
Pack a 1 pint wide mouth mason jar with 1 oz arnica leaf and 4 oz almond oil and put on lid. Stir or shake daily for 2-3 weeks. Strain.
*To make balm. Heat beeswax until melted. Combine the arnica infused oil with melted beeswax, stir well. Add Vitamin E, stir again and Pour into jars with tight fitting lids. Makes about 7 oz = 7 (1 oz) jars or 14 (1/2oz) Jars

CAYENNE MINT SALVE
Used for pain and inflammation. Great for back and muscle pain.
1 cayenne pepper cut and diced (Use gloves and remove the seeds)
1/4 cup fresh mint
1/3 cup olive oil
Put in a container and shake. Let steep for 7 hours.
Then add the ingredients below. Melt the cocoa butter and beeswax in the microwave in 30 second increments until melted.
4 oz cocoa butter (Melted)
2 oz bees wax. (Melted)
Mix well and put into a salve jar. Makes 7-8 oz

GRAPEVINE SAP SALVE
Used for skin diseases
1/4 cup grape vine sap (see below)

2 oz cocoa butter
1 oz beeswax
1 teaspoon Vitamin E
Put fresh plump grape vines through a noodle press (collecting the sap from inside) set a side. Heat cocoa butter and bees wax until melted. Add sap and vitamin E. take off heat, stir for a minute or two so it is mixed well and put into a clean dry glass salve container. Makes 4 oz

HORSE CHESTNUT SALVE
Use for sore muscles and leg cramps
1 horse chestnut fruit crushed
1 tablespoon carrier oil
4 tablespoons cocoa butter
Mix crushed fruit and put in carrier oil and allow to sit in the sun 1 day. Next day strain the oil making sure to get all the oil by pushing it into the strainer. Heat cocoa butter to liquid and mix in the oil and put into a salve jar. Makes about 1.5 oz

LEMON-MINT PAIN SALVE
For pain from muscles
1 cup fresh lemon mint leaves
3/4 cup carrier oil (I like sweet almond oil)
Bruise leaves and combine with carrier oil in a pan on warm (the notch just before low), sauté for 1 hour, cool, and strain. This can be done on the stove or the slow cooker.
4 oz cocoa butter
2 oz bees wax
Mix beeswax with cocoa butter and melt. Add infused oil from above and mix well. Pour into sterilized jars. Makes approximately 12 oz / three 4 oz jars / six 2 oz jars

SLIPPERY ELM DRAWING SALVE (for boils)
1 tablespoon slippery elm powder (or make your own by pulverizing dried slippery elm bark)
3 drops tea tree E.O.
2 drops Lavender E.O. Or Thyme E.O.
Mix together the above and make a paste (add a drop or two of distilled water if needed) and apply to the boil after using a hot compress for 10 minutes. Cover loosely with a dressing for 24 hours.

ANTIBIOTIC OINTMENT
This salve is great for diaper rash and dry skin in winter, besides healing cuts and scrapes.
4 oz extra virgin olive oil

1/4 oz dried calendula (marigold) flowers
1/4 oz dried thyme leaves
1/4 oz dried peppermint leaves
1/4 oz lavender flowers
4 oz beeswax
4 oz coconut oil
In a 1 qt mason jar add calendula, thyme, peppermint and lavender. Put in the olive oil and let sit for 14 days. Then, strain the mixture reserving the infused oil. In a medium saucepan or microwave combine the coconut oil and bees wax until melted. Add the infused oil mixing well and pour into small jars. Close top after salve has cooled.

ATHLETES FOOT OINTMENT
You know what this is for
2 oz sweet almond oil
1 oz cocoa butter or Shea butter
10 drops tea tree EO
8 drops Lavender EO
8 drops peppermint EO
Melt the cocoa butter then add the rest. Mix well and store in a opaque glass jar. To use apply to affected area
~ LIP BALMS ~

LEMON UP LIP BALM
A wonderful healing blend and kids love it
1 tablespoon cocoa butter
1 teaspoon beeswax
1/4 teaspoon vitamin E
6 drops lemon essential oil
Melt cocoa butter and bees wax add the rest and stir well. Put in a lip balm container. A kids favorite.
VARIATIONS could include replacing the lemon EO with Cotton candy fragrance oil, strawberry fragrance oil, Or monkey farts fragrance oil for boys.

CINNAMON LIP BALM
The sweet spicy that everyone will love
1 tablespoon cocoa butter
1 teaspoon bees wax
1/4 teaspoon vitamin E
2 drops cinnamon essential oil
Heat cocoa butter and beeswax until melted. Then add the vitamin E and essential oil and stir well. Put in a lip balm container. A favorite among teens.

VARIATIONS could include Peppermint EO in place of cinnamon EO or a fragrance oil like mocha cappuccino, Pina Colada fragrance oil, or Chocolate strawberries fragrance oil.

LEMON BALM COLD SORE LIP BALM #1
Has a nice lemon mint fragrance and a cooling effect on the area. Makes a nice chap stick also.
1/2 teaspoon lemon balm infused oil or 8 drops Lemon Balm EO
1/2 teaspoon peppermint infused oil or 8 Drops Peppermint EO
1 oz cocoa butter
1 oz bees wax
Melt cocoa butter and bees wax, add the infused oils or Essential oils and mix well. Pour into lip stick tubes and allow to set. Cap and use as needed.

Bayberry Lip balm
These go really well at craft fairs around the winter holiday's and are enjoyed by men, women and children
1 tablespoon bayberry wax (see chapter 13 to make wax)
2 tablespoons cocoa butter
1 vitamin E tab (400 IU)
Melt wax and cocoa butter in a glass measuring cup in the microwave for 15 second increments until melted. Add vitamin E tab by piercing the tab and squeezing out the oil. Mix well. Pour into either lip

LEMON BALM -MINT LIP BALM OR SALVE #2
For cold sores (herpes virus)
You will need 1 oz of lemon balm - mint tincture (made with sweet almond oil) from chapter 8
1 oz beeswax
1 oz cocoa butter (100%)
Heat the bees wax and cocoa butter until liquid watching closely. Take off heat or from microwave. Add the tincture stir well and pour into small salve jars or into lip balm tubes. Allow to cool and harden before capping. To use simply apply to your lips.

PEPPERMINT – THYME BALM
For cold sores(herpes) or as a joint-muscle pain and inflammation salve
This can be made into a lip balm or used as a salve on genital Herpes as well as a inflamed muscle and joint salve
4 oz cocoa butter
2 oz olive oil (infused with 1/2 oz each of thyme and peppermint.

1/2 teaspoon Vitamin E
Put thyme and peppermint into a small glass jar and add olive oil. Let sit 14 days and strain. Melt the coconut butter then add the infused oil and vitamin E. Mix well and put into Salve jars or lip balm containers. Makes 6 oz.

~ HERBAL POULTICES ~

A poultice is a crushed herb, flowers or root and is applied to an affected area

ARNICA POULTICE
3 tablespoons flowers in a cup of hot water. Let stand 10 minutes and apply plant material to injury for 15 minutes. Repeat 3-4 times daily for acute injury.

BURDOCK ROOT POULTICE
crushed or grated fresh root is used for sores and bug bites

CHAMOMILE POPPY POULTICE
For pain relief
Mix equal amount of poppy heads and chamomile flowers. Then soak them in hot water for 5 minutes. Then apply to area of pain. Leave on 30 minutes and repeat as needed.

CALENDULA POULTICE OR COMPRESS (2 for 1)
Can use the liquid as a compress liquid and the plant material as a poultice.
2 teaspoons calendula flowers
1 cup hot water
Steep 10 minutes, strain out plant material and use as a poultice and use liquid cooled as a compress.

GRAPE LEAF POULTICE
Used to stop bleeding, reduce inflammation.
Grape leaves are torn into small pieces and put in hot water for a few minutes then placed on a wound.
Leave there 10-25 minutes and replace if needed.

GINGER ROOT POULTICE (crushed fresh root)
for burns (relieves the pain instantly)
Grate fresh or died ginger root and pour a little bit of hot water over for
5 minutes and then, Drain and put on burn.

YARROW POULTICE
crushed leaves, flowers and whole plant) for swollen joints, cuts,
wounds.
Put crushed leaves in a little hot water for a few minutes then strain and
use plant material on wound.
*Can Chew leaves to relieve toothaches.

CHAPTER 12 VARIOUS USES FOR COMMON ITEMS

ALOE - You can grow this in a kitchen window. If you buy the gel make sure it is Aloin free.
*Type 2 diabetics take 10-20 ml of gel inside leaf(about 1 tablespoon) two times a day to regulate blood sugar levels.
**For colitis 25-30 ml (about two tablespoons) of gel inside leaf two times a day.
*** For burns or sunburn apply several times a day until skin returns to normal.
****To soften skin use as often as needed.
*****For scrapes and minor cuts use as needed. Not for open wounds or surgery wounds.

APPLE CIDER VINEGAR
*for Heavy dandruff - pour on the apple cider vinegar let sit 2-5 minutes and rinse well. Will also make your hair soft.
** for scabies, spider mites or other microscopic crawlies on skin - pour on the apple cider vinegar let sit 5 minutes and rinse.

ANGELINA - Can be smoked like tobacco

ARNICA (Arnica Montana) is grown in all parts of the US and will grow in cool climates, poor and often acidic soil and in mountains. Can buy in any seed store. But there are 26 different genus. Use in creams, gels , essential oil and salves. Should NOT be used on open wounds or broken skin.
*A wonderful pain relieving rub that invigorates circulation

Bee stings apply meat tenderizer mixed with a bit of water to make a paste, it will stop the allergic
 reaction. Keep it on hand when camping.

Bergamot is Earl Grey tea Use the leaves to make tea.

Cats Claw protects against (NSAID) like ibuprofen's gastrointestinal damage. Is a compliment to cancer treatments, and has been used for HIV and AIDS

CAYENNE - stimulate stomach lining cells to secrete a substance that prevents ulcers.
*It also helps regulate blood sugar levels by breaking down carbohydrates after a meal.
**Use in salves to give pain relieving heat.

CHAMOMILE - used in a mouth wash has been proven to prevent mouth sores associated with chemotherapy and radiation.

CHICKWEED - Cook the young stems and eat like spinach. Chickweed is both an oil and an acid and
 can be taken both internally and externally for Skin diseases. Amazing as asthma relief.

CORNSTARCH Apply to Athletes feet with a few drops Peppermint EO before putting into socks in the morning

ECHINACEA – using the juice from the root on your skin makes the fiery heat of a sweat lodge more tolerable.
*It also heals burns and wounds.
** Chew the leaves and root for tooth aches, sore gums and sore throat.

FENNEL SEEDS -chewed will dull hunger pangs. 1 teaspoon fennel seeds, 1 cup boiling water let steep 10 minutes and strain. Cool before diluting it in half for an infant. Use as it for an adult.
*A tea has been recommended for colicky infants.
**It also stimulates breast milk in lactating women.

FEVERFEW- Chew 1/2 -1 small leaf a day to wart off headaches. (If mouth ulcers start discontinue use and it will clear up)
**chew 2 leaves if having a migraine.

GINGER POWDERED RHIZONE ROOT - taken for general emetic a single does of 1-2 g, for motion sickness take 2-4 daily

GRAPES - are eaten for kidney and liver diseases, cholera, and cancer

GRAPE LEAF -used as a poultice to stop bleeding and reduce swelling. (See recipe under Chapter 11)

HYSSOP – should not be taken if pregnant

HOPS -for toothache pain.
*Make a tea, decoction, or poultice. 1 Cup Fresh
** Died hops put in a small draw string bag and put in your pillow case will give you a restful sleep.

HORSE CHECTNUT -dried powdered seed dose is 1-2 g a day for Chronic venous insufficiency

JUNIPER BERRIES - are chewed to stimulate appetite and relieve indigestion.
*To apply to skin use 10 drops essential oil in 1 oz carrier oil.]
**For other ailments take 1-2 g died berries three times a day

Kelp- has been used after radiation
* is useful when taking x-rays

MULLEIN TEA - from leaves and flowers is used for expectorant, coughs, and throat related ills.
*Smoking the leaves for respiratory distress, bronchitis, asthma or can ingest an infusion.

MAYONNAISE- will KILL LICE, it will also condition your hair. Lather up your entire body, head to toe and leave on 30 minutes.

Nettle for hair loss and prostate. 1 tablespoon nettle, 1 cup hot water, steep 10 minutes and strain.
NOTE:Use as compress or infusion. Make a compress for prostate. Make a infusion for hair.

PEPPERMINT - mixed with salt for dog bites and rabies- Crush leaves, and moisten with small amount of hot water. Let sit 10 minutes, Add salt and apply to wound, cover with a bandage, replace two or more times a day (morning and night)

PSYLLIUM- Take 2-3 tablespoons of seeds a day. Half before breakfast and half before dinner for lowering (LDL) cholesterol, irritable bowel syndrome, as a laxative OR weight control.
*Kids take 1 teaspoon divided between breakfast and dinner.
NOTE: Make sure you take enough water. These hold ten times their weight in water. Consult Doctor before taking if you have had bowel surgery.

SAW PALMETTO - take 160 milligrams twice a day. The dried berry stops the hormone BHP from attacking the prostate gland and it acts as an anti-inflammatory. And it works better than "Proscar" without the side effects.

SLIPPERY ELM- for inflammation. Mix 2 tablespoons powdered bark with 1/4 cup water(add a little more if needed to mix completely. Apply to inflamed area on skin for 20-30 minutes reapply as needed.

TUMERIC - Sundry the rhizomes. To use take 1.5 to 3 g dried root daily for your liver and to aid in digestion of fats which will help an ailing gall bladder

CHAPTER 13 CREATING ON A BUDGET

There comes a time in everyones life when money just isn't flowing like we need. It is at those times that we need to be our most resourceful. The following recipes are created with backyard herbs and the dollar store finds. These are found at either the Family Dollar and Dollar General stores. You will need these items!

Family Dollar's " Vitamin E 4,000 I.U. Skin oil" (4 oz) Usually $1.5- $2. (Both stores have a Vitamin E) NOTE: cheapest at Family Dollar. Can be used in any of the recipes in this book that calls for vitamin E

Cocoa butter (1 oz) (push up container) Usually $1 Family Dollar You can use in any cocoa butter recipe found in this book. This size is wonderful for many of the recipes.

Nadinola Cocoa Butter Cream (4 oz) Usually $1.25-$1.50 Use the creamy one in the Queens hand lotion recipe NOTE: I prefer this one to the Dollar General version.

Nadinola Cocoa Butter (4 oz) Usually $1.50-$2 in a white plastic jar with a brown lid at family Dollar store (Check inside because sometimes in the same jar it is a cream instead of cocoa butter) The solid one you can use in any cocoa butter recipe found in this book. NOTE: I prefer this one to the Dollar General version

Queen Helene Cocoa butter crème at Dollar General(4.8 oz) opaque jar Usually $1.50 (check inside - one will look like a creamy body butter and the other a greasy solid. But check as both are marked the same but are completely different once you open the jars (what is up with that?) Use the creamy one for Queens hand lotion. The solid one you can use in the recipes below only.

Witch hazel 16 oz bottle Usually $1-$1.25 Both stores. NOTE: for some reason family dollar only has the 71% mix Witch hazel.

Rubbing alcohol 16 oz bottle (91%) Usually $1.50-$2 it is in a squared bottle. The round ones have (71%) Dollar General.

~RECIPES WITH WITCH HAZEL ~

CALENDULA – WITCH HAZEL WOUND LOTION
Used for dermatitis, wounds, skin problems, eczema, abscesses, acne, skin abrasions, wounds, to kill bacteria.
8 oz witch hazel (1/2 container)
2 oz calendula flowers (from garden also known as pot marigold)
In a 1 qt mason jar put both the herb and the witch hazel and steep for 14 days. Strain and pour into a glass jar with a tight fitting lid or back into the container you bought it in. To use put some on a cotton ball and put on affected area.

THYME-WITCH HAZEL ACNE CLEANSER
Works well on cleaning cuts and scrapes. Thyme cleans, is an antibiotic and reduces swelling of trouble acne, or swollen cuts and good on Eczema, varicose veins
8 oz witch hazel (1/2 container)
2 oz thyme leaves (from garden)
In a 1 qt mason jar put both the herb and the witch hazel and steep for 14 days. Strain and pour into a glass jar with a tight fitting lid or back into the container you bought it in. To use put some on a cotton ball and put on affected area.

PAIN RELEIVING PEPPERMINT-WITCH HAZEL ACNE CLEANSER
Also works well on cleaning cuts and scrapes. Peppermint also relieves the pain.
8 oz witch hazel (1/2 container)
2 oz peppermint leaves (from garden)
In a 1 qt mason jar put both the herb and the witch hazel and steep for 14 days. Strain and pour into a glass jar with a tight fitting lid or back into the container you bought it in. To use put some on a cotton ball and put on affected area.

MILK THISTLE-WITCH HAZEL PSORIASIS LOTION

This one is wonderful for psoriasis.
8 oz witch hazel (1/2 container)
2 oz milk thistle flowers(from back yard or woodland area)
In a 1 qt mason jar put both the herb and the witch hazel and steep for 14 days. Strain and pour into a glass jar with a tight fitting lid or back into the container you bought it in. To use put some on a cotton ball and put on affected area.

~ QUEEN HELENE COCOA BUTTER CREME ~ (the creamy one)

QUEENS HAND LOTION
Just a wonderful scented hard working hand lotion
1 jar Queen Helene Cocoa Butter crème Or Nadinola Cocoa Butter Cream (the soft fluffy -creamy one)
1 teaspoons vitamin E
1/3 cup distilled water (maybe more)
1 teaspoon Almond extract, vanilla extract, or lemon extract (from the spice dept at same store)*
In a mixing bowl put in the cocoa butter crème, the vitamin E and the extract of your choosing. With a mixer beat on low speed. Add water a little at a time until all is incorporated. Add more water if desired. I use old liquid soap containers to put the lotion in.

DESIGNER QUEENS HAND LOTION
You pick the scent hand lotion
1 jar Queen Helene Cocoa Butter crème Or Nadinola Cocoa Butter Cream (the soft fluffy -creamy one)
1 teaspoons vitamin E
1/3 cup distilled water (maybe more)
1/2 teaspoon any of their fake designer perfume scents at front of store at checkout $1-$2
In a mixing bowl put in the cocoa butter crème, the vitamin E and the fake designer perfume of your choosing. With a mixer beat on low speed. Add water a little at a time until all is incorporated. Add more water if desired. I use old liquid soap containers to put the lotion in.

~ QUEEN HELENE COCOA BUTTER CREME ~(the greasy one)

QUEENS PAIN SALVE
This is great for any pain.
1 jar Queen Helene Cocoa Butter Creme (the greasy solid one)
1 oz Peppermint leaves (garden) or Willow bark (Back yard) that has
been put through a coffee grinder. Heat cocoa butter crème on warm on
the stove (or mini crock pot on warm) add the peppermint and stir. Cook
on warm for 2-4 hours. Strain and put into a salve jar.

QUEENS PAIN AND SWELLING SALVE (The greasy one)
This is great for any pain that is accompanied with swelling.
1 jar Queen Helene Cocoa butter Creme (the greasy solid one)
1/2 oz thyme leaves (garden)
1/2 oz Peppermint leaves (Garden)or Willow bark* (Back yard)(*put
through a coffee grinder).
Heat cocoa butter crème on warm on the stove (or mini crock pot on
warm) add the peppermint and thyme and stir. Cook on warm for 2-4
hours. Strain and put into a salve jar.

QUEENS ARTHRITIS SALVE (The greasy one)
For the Arthritis suffer
1 jar Queen Helene Cocoa butter Creme (the greasy solid one)
1 oz burdock (from back yard or woodland area)
Heat cocoa butter crème on warm on the stove (or mini crock pot on
warm) add the burdock and stir. Cook on warm for 2-4 hours. Strain and
put into a salve jar. This can be applied two ways. Rub into arthritic
body parts or heat a small amount back to liquid, cool slightly and apply
warm but not too hot liquid salve to arthritic joints, hands, ect.

QUEENS PSORIASIS SALVE (The greasy one)
This is great for Psoriasis.
1 jar Queen Helene Cocoa butter Creme (the greasy solid one)
1 oz Milk thistle flowers put through a coffee grinder.
Heat cocoa butter crème on warm on the stove (or mini crock pot on
warm) add the milk thistle and stir. Cook on warm for 2-4 hours. Strain
and put into a salve jar. Apply to any psoriasis patch and gently rub in.

QUEENS MULTI-USE SALVE (The greasy one)
For bruises, sprains, and wounds
1 jar Queen Helene Cocoa butter Creme (the greasy solid one)
1 oz elder leaves.

Heat cocoa butter crème on warm on the stove (or mini crock pot on warm) add the elder leaves and stir. Cook on warm for 2-4 hours. Strain and put into a salve jar. Use on bruises, sprains and wounds.

QUEENS RHEUMATISM SALVE (The greasy one)
For Aches and pains from Rheumatism
1 jar Queen Helene Cocoa butter Creme (the greasy solid one)
1 oz elder flowers.
Heat cocoa butter crème on warm on the stove (or mini crock pot on warm) add the elder flowers and stir. Cook on warm for 2-4 hours. Strain and put into a salve jar. Rub the salve over achy joints.

~ RUBBING ALCOHOL RECIPES ~

PEPPERMIN T MASSAGE RUB
Relieves tired, achy muscles, achy feet, and since peppermint is anti-fungal it will sooth athletes foot.
8 oz rubbing alcohol
2 oz peppermint from the garden
In a 1 qt mason jar put both the herb and rubbing alcohol. Steep for 14 days. Strain and pour into spray bottle. To use spray some on your sore back or other muscle and massage in.

BURDOCK ARTHRITIS RELIEF
For arthritis pain
8 oz rubbing alcohol
2 oz burdock (from the woods)
In a 1 qt mason jar put both the herb and rubbing alcohol. Steep for 14 days. Strain and pour into a glass jar or back into container it was bought in. To use apply with a cotton ball or rub in with hands.

~100% Cocoa butter ~

100% Cocoa butter in white jar or push up stick can be used in any of the recipes anywhere in this book that calls for cocoa butter, Salves, lip balms, and ointments. *
If using Queen Helene in the opaque container, the one made from (cocoa seed) it has more oils so stick to the recipes above.

~Vitamin E ~

The vitamin E found there can be used on any recipe needing vitamin e

Bayberry Wax
Make your own Bayberry Wax for candles and soaps. You can even use in your lotions and balms. You will need access to either a bayberry bush or a wax myrtle bush (Myria cerifera). Pick the berries in November and put them in a large pot with water equal to the amount of berries.
Bring to a boil and simmer until thick and syrupy. Strain the berries and seeds from the syrup and cool in a heat proof bowl. When cool and it solidifies you can pick the wax off the top. Store in an air tight container until you have enough for your project. After you make the wax here is a quick little lip balm you can make with the wax